Spirituality and Healing

A Multicultural Perspective

Spirituality and Healing

A Multicultural Perspective

Wynne DuBray, Editor

Writers Club Press

San Jose New York Lincoln Shanghai

Spirituality and Healing
A Multicultural Perspective

Writers Club Press
an imprint of iUniverse, Inc.

For information address:
iUniverse, Inc.
5220 S. 16th St., Suite 200
Lincoln, NE 68512
www.iuniverse.com

ISBN: 0-595-20607-7

Printed in the United States of America

Preface

During the last twenty-five years, I have been teaching multicultural content in Schools of Social Work to both graduate and undergraduate students. As I have studied the different populations in our society, I became aware of the importance of *spirituality* in the lives and world views of representatives of each group. Usually, this was associated with the healing of the mind, body, and spirit of the people.

Ceremonies and rituals continue to play an important part in these societies today, as do their spiritual leaders. For some societies, it was the one unifying force, which contributed to their survival, as they faced oppressive invasion of their communities, families, and personal lives by government officials. Laws were passed in the United States forbidding the native people from practicing their centuries old traditions and ceremonies, yet, the spiritual practices continued in secret. Their healing practices continued because it was the very foundation of their societies.

Social work, as a profession, is beginning to acknowledge the importance of spirituality in working with clients suffering from terminal illnesses, family breakup, trauma, alienation, depression, addictions, and a multitude of other problems. As social workers acknowledge and examine their own spiritual perspectives, they become aware of a very basic need in our society. In fact, there appears to be a spiritual vacuum in our society, which is not being met by the organized religious institutions. A challenge for social workers, and other human service personnel, is to open up the spiritual aspects of peoples' lives that remain, far too often, closed off from family, friends, and professionals in human service. Once these aspects are open, another challenge for social workers is to understand spirituality in the context of the individual's overall biopsychosocial profile, and to consider spirituality as a possible vehicle to facilitate growth and change in the individual.

This text attempts to address these challenges and exposes the practitioner to interventions which can have a healing effect on the mind, body, and spirit of ourselves and our clients. It is hoped that this text will enhance the services delivered to multicultural populations and enhance the lives of the practitioners, as well. The support and wisdom of numerous people have contributed to this book. Institutional assistance in the form of a sabbatical leave from California State University, Sacramento was especially appreciated. The contributions of Josè Guadalupe, Santos Torres, Marietta Rubien, Peter Navarro, Adelle Sanders, and Sarah Rose greatly enhanced this text.

My own ideas were particularly influenced by my parents, Peter and Lillian DuBray, who have long since joined the spirit world. Other great teachers were the thousands of clients, students, friends, and family members who have shared their spiritual lives with me throughout my life as a daughter, wife, grandmother, mother, sister, mentor, practitioner, and friend to many.

We are spiritual beings with physical experiences!
Wynne DuBray

Acknowledgments

Spirituality and Healing: A Multicultural Perspective represents a collaborative undertaking of friends and colleagues from different ethnicities and backgrounds. Reflecting upon our own cultural heritage and our own experiences with religious and spiritual activities and the experiences of our friends and clients has been a blessing for each of us.

We wish to thank our families and friends, who have supported us in our interest and commitment in providing culturally sensitive and competent services over many years. Their patience was also appreciated as we undertook the research for and writing of this book.
Wynne DuBray and Associates

Cover design by Wynne DuBray, Lakota Artist
The cover design, of a feather, symbolizes prayer and spiritual communication with the *Great Mystery* of the Lakota Nation.

Contents

Introduction

As professional human service workers, we are constantly reflecting upon our work and our effectiveness. Are we helping or harming those we seek to serve? Are we sensitive to the needs of our clients? Can we provide what our clients need? Are we involved in cultural malpractice? Do we make an effort to understand the diverse cultural backgrounds of our clients and the impact that culture has had on their lives? Are we aware of the part that spirituality and religion play in the development of the personalities of both ourselves and our clients?

There was a time, in the not too distant past, that to mention spirituality in the context of assessment and services was not appropriate. Although most of us realized that spirituality was an important part of human behavior and personality development, we were reluctant to bring it out in the open for fear of being criticized by our peers. Today, spirituality is being addressed in professional educational programs of psychology and social work. It is seen as a valuable and basic part of our human existence. Techniques of spiritual assessment have been published in recent textbooks. Seminars are offered in the social work profession and in psychology to assist practitioners in understanding the connection between spirituality and healing.

Spirituality is closely connected to cultural teachings. How spirituality is defined and experienced is guided by cultural traditions and religious doctrine. A *Lakota* child watches her father pray to the four directions, as he rises at sunrise and faces the east holding an eagle feather or the sacred pipe in his outstretched hand held upward. Spirituality to this family is defined as the *Great Mystery*, which is everywhere at all times. Therefore, it is important to pray to the four directions of the universe, to give thanks for each new day. Life is seen as a precious gift.

The Buddhist asks the imaginary bird on his left shoulder, "what will this day bring?" The Catholic holds the beads of the rosary as she or he prays to Jehovah. The recovering addict puts trust in a higher power to assist in overcoming a life threatening condition. Each experiences the spirit in his or her own way and gains strength from this connection.

Within each culture, individuals are at different stages of assimilation and adaptation to their environment. Definitions and perceptions of spirituality and healing change as the person grows and experiences life. Some Indigenous people may embrace Christianity, but others may practice the traditions of their people that have existed for centuries.

The United States becomes more diverse each day, as new immigrants arrive with their cultural traditions and healing practices. We, as human service workers, must become more accepting and sophisticated in understanding the many and diverse perspectives of spirituality. With spiritual traditions comes healing practices, which differs from Western medicine. Today, alternative methods of healing are becoming popular and even accepted by Health Maintenance Organizations.

Everyone has heard of the placebo effect which is based upon the power of the belief system within the psyche. Belief systems, prayer, and other spiritual practices play a prominent role in our healing. Healing permeates the spiritual, emotional, and physical aspects of human existence and brings a sense of wholeness to the individual.

It is because of this need for spiritual awareness on the part of human service workers that this text was written. Many human service workers are overworked, with large caseloads and a limited amount of time to do research on cultural groups. This text provides a concise, easy to read handbook to assist the culturally sensitive practitioner with needed information regarding multicultural aspects of spirituality and healing. This text addresses the tip of the iceberg, and it is by no means a comprehensive review of the subject. If it serves as a catalyst for more culturally competent services, it will have fulfilled its purpose.

On a new path we walk...

Wynne DuBray

Chapter 1

American Indian Spirituality and Healing Practices

Wynne DuBray

To write a chapter on American Indian healing practices is an awesome task, to say the least. With the hundreds of tribes, each with different ceremonies and interpretations, the task seems overwhelming. There is great diversity among Indian people tribally, regionally, historically, and politically. Yet, it is possible to draw some similarities amongst tribal ceremonies and describe some of those common to more than one tribe (DuBray, 2000).

Although the philosophies and spiritual practices of each American Indian group or tribe are different, there is a thread of consistency, or a sameness, among these practices. Each American Indian group has its own tribal mythology, or cosmology, which describes its origin, explains the genesis of the cosmos, including the earth in its myriad of live forms, and provides models for modern behavior. Mythology, or cosmology, is a mirror of and a map for the culture that believes in and practices it. Therefore, mythology may be defined as a great body of truth for the people who believe. Mythology explains the relationship of the people to the cosmos. Some people prefer the word cosmology to the term mythology. Having respect and love for life, the Creator of life, and those that have lived before, are important features of American Indian spirituality. The whole religion is like a preparation or path to the *good land*, or the path of

1

the ancestors. All have to go through it. Each day American Indian people thank the Creator for this life.

American Indians know that they can never leave *nature*, as it is a part of them, and they are a part of nature. When the Indian stands in the early dawn praying to the Great Spirit (the great mystery) in humility, it is an acknowledgment of the importance of being and staying in balance and in harmony with nature. The great mystery, or life force, is acknowledged in all creatures of nature, including the rocks and mountains (DuBray, 2000).

This emphasis on *balance* is central to all tribal spiritual practices. *Balance* is another way of viewing harmony with one's environment, whether it be family, friends, community, work place, school, or the animal kingdom. This leads to respect for nature and all living creatures. Rocks and rivers are considered living entities and, therefore, are respected. Animals taken for food are considered sacred and are thanked and blessed before taking their life for consumption (DuBray, 1999).

American Indians place great value on the symbiotic relationship between themselves and the earth. Allen (1999) explains, "We are the land. More than remembered, the Earth is the mind of the people as we are the mind of the earth. The land is not an image in our eyes but rather it is as truly an integral aspect of our being as we are of its being" (Allen as cited in Trout, 1999,p. 10). The inter- relatedness between people and the place they live is seen as a complete organism. Everything affects everything else. To understand them, it is necessary to see into their complexity. This organism includes the living, as well as the inert, as seen in American Indian stories describing the Earth Mother and the Sky Father. The oral literatures of numerous American Indian groups pair the earth with the sky. Frequently, they are addressed as 'mother' and 'father' to express a family connection among parts of the visible universe (Trout, 1999).

Environmental Issues

American Indians know how to take excellent care of the earth, unlike the dominant segment of society. Few generalizations cover all of their philosophies, but there are basic points that are relevant when contemplating the future of this plane and its limited resources. The tribes, representing various civilizations, ultimately understood their relationship with their environments (Fixico, 1998). The rest of the world is finally becoming aware of the fragility of the earth and the finiteness of natural resources. American Indians are challenged with the task of preserving the environment while at the same time strengthening their sovereignty.

Another concept common to tribes is the *circle*. The *circle* has spiritual connotations of healing. The *circle of life* is a view of life from infancy to death as a circle. Many tribes believe in reincarnation, thus the circle continues as the spirit re-incarnates again in another human body. All ceremonies are conducted in a circle. There are *prayer circles* and *talking circles,* which are powerful spiritual healing experiences. Many Indians originally lived in circular lodges, tepees, huts, and hogans. The California Indians conducted their healing ceremonies in the *round houses*, which were mostly underground with an opening in the center to let in the light beams of the sun. The Lakotas believe that the Great Spirit is blessing a gathering of people when the great bald eagle circles over the group three times.

The *medicine wheel* is another example of the circle symbolism in healing. The *medicine wheel* is a round circle with the four directions superimposed upon it. This is an ancient symbol used by almost all the Native people of North America and South America. There are many different ways that this basic concept is expressed: the four directions of North , East, South and West, starting at the top of the circle and going clockwise is one of the most common methods. The North point represents mental processes, the East represents the spiritual processes, the South represents the emotions, and the West represents the physical parts of life (DuBray, 2000).

The number four repeats as an important number among American Indian tribes. Other examples of the use of the number four are the four *symbolic races* (Black, White, Red, andYellow). There are four *physical world elements* (water, fire, earth, and air). There are four *worlds of existence* (mineral, animal, human, and plant/vegetable). In addition, there are four *dimensions of human knowledge* (understanding, action, reflection, and interpretation).

Four has many important meanings to the Lakota, as well as to many other tribes. There are *four ages*: the age of the child; the age of adolescent; the age of the adult; and, the age of the aged. There are four *things that breathe*: those that crawl; those that fly; those that are two-legged; and, those that are four-legged. There are four *things above the earth*: sun; moon; stars; and, planets. There are four *parts to the green things*: roots; stem; leaves; and, fruit. There are four *divisions of time*: day; night; moon; and, year.

The Indian strives to express, in ceremony and in symbology, a reflection of four: There are four *endurances* in the Sweat Lodge, four *direction offerings* in the Pipe Ceremony, and four *direction facings* in the Sun Dance. The vision quester carries four colors and places these four colors in a square within which he or she sits. Other references to the number four are the four grandfathers, the four winds, the four cardinal directions, and many other relationships that can be expressed in sets of four. Just like a mirror can be used to see things not normally seen (e.g., behind us or around a corner), the *medicine wheel* can be used to help us see or understand things we cannot quite see or understand because they are ideas and not physical objects.

A *relational* worldview, sometimes called the *cyclical world view*, is common to tribal cultures. It is non-time oriented, fluid, and intuitive. Balance and harmony in all relationships is the foundation of this philosophy, which includes interaction with spiritual forces. Human service workers are viewed as healers who can assist an individual in reestablishing balance among many interrelating factors in one's circle of life. Health exists only when all elements are in balance or harmony. Helpers and healers, upon entering the world of the client, manipulate the balance contextually, cognitively, emotionally, physically, and/or spiritually. An effective helper is one who has an understanding of the complex, interdependent nature of life and can utilize physical, psychological, contextual, and spiritual forces to promote harmony and balance.(Red Voices,2000).

Concepts of power and relationships for the Lakota include all life dimensions. Gaining or developing power, one definition of empowerment (Cox & Parsons, 1994), is viewed by the Lakota as receiving help from the spiritual and natural world for a higher purpose than the individual self. This assistance is to benefit the entire Lakota Nation.

Lakota Ceremonies

Among the Lakota people, there are a number of important ceremonies that one must become familiar with, when working with Lakota people. These traditional ceremonies are explained in this section. They include, *Keeping of the Soul, Inipi: The Sweat Lodge Ceremony or Rite of Purification, Hanblecheyapi: Vision Quest, Wiwanyag Wachipi: The Sundance Ceremony, Hankapi: Making Relatives, Ishnata Awicalowan: Preparing A Girl for Womanhood*, and *Tapa Wanka Yap: Throwing the Ball*. All of these ceremonies have a healing effect on the participants and are manifestations of the spiritual life of the individuals as it relates to the family, group, and community (McGaa, 1989).

Keeping of the Soul:

In the Lakota tradition, this was the first rite of seven given by the White Buffalo Calf Woman to the people. In this ceremony, the soul of a dead loved one is purified so it can return to the Great Spirit. The second part of the ceremony is the give-away, which takes place a year after death. All of the deceased's possessions are given away a year after the funeral. During the year, the widow or widower makes and procures gifts and decides what friends will be the recipients. The gifts are presented at a give-away dinner. It is a wonderful non-materialistic activity in the remembrance of a departed relative or friend (McGaa, 1989).

Inipi: The Sweat Lodge Ceremony or Rite of Purification:

While people of the world are struggling with spirituality, spirituality has forever been an integral part of life for the American Indian; yet, the complexities of modern Western culture make observing a spiritual way increasingly difficult. The sweat ceremony is at the heart of the spiritual life of most American Indians.

This ceremony is used as a cleansing ceremony. It is part of healing and restoration. It is the mending of a broken connection between people. The participants in a ceremony say the words "all my relations' *Mitake Oyasin*", before and after the prayer. These words create a relationship between humans, animals, and the land. To have health, it is necessary to keep all those relations in mind. The intention of this ceremony is to purify and heal the spirit. This healing is accomplished by a kind of inner cleansing of the inner self and a geography of the human spirit and the rest of the world. The broken off pieces of self and the world are reunited and become whole again. Each person brings together the fragments of their lives in a sacred act of renewal, and connections are re-established with others.

This ceremony requires a structure, fire, and water. It represents the universe and connects the participants to the past, the earth, and the spiritual world. It is a place for teaching, praying, singing, purifying, and communing with others. As participants sing, pray, and enter into a trance, they believe that the ritual sweat bath purges their impurities and brings both spiritual and physical health by restoring balance. One feels renewed, reborn, and purified after participation in the ceremony. Women and men usually have separate ceremonies. Most of the American Indian residential alcohol treatment programs throughout the nation incorporate this ceremony in their programs to enhance the recovery of participants, regardless of their tribal affiliation.

Hanblecheyapi: Vision Quest:

This ceremony is performed on an isolated mountain top or butte and places the quester alone before the Great Mystery. The vision seeker endures a period of fasting and going without water. The vision quester prepares himself or herself in the sweat lodge before ascending to the isolated area. In cool weather or at higher elevations, a blanket or a sleeping bag is needed. This ceremony requires only the quester and four twigs with pieces of colored cloth, representing the four directions, tied to them. This is an especially important ceremony for young people who are ready to face the challenges of the adult world. It is a time of reflection on their spiritual and occupational paths (McGaa,1989).

The purpose of the *vision quest* is not to make one's self feel important or to be interesting to one's friends, but to realize the vastness of the universe and the oneness with it. The *vision quest* is done for the purpose of self-improvement. It is done for a deeper insight into the why of one's being here.

Wiwanyag Wachipi: The Sun Dance Ceremony:

The Sun Dance is the annual coming together of the tribe to thank the Great Spirit for all that has been given to the people. The emphasis is on tribal unity, peace, and strength through the honor and thanksgiving offered to the Great Spirit. This ceremony lasts for four days and is usually held in late July or early August. It begins on a Thursday and ends on a Sunday. The ceremony requires a cotton wood tree, an arena, and a tribal gathering. The Sun Dance chief is usually the most respected holy man among the medicine people and one who is very knowledgeable in the traditions of the Lakota. He is responsible for the ceremonial activities and makes most major decisions during the four day event.

The men wear a kilt skirt secured by a belt around the waist, or use a woman's shawl as a dance kilt. Sage wreaths circle the dancers' wrists and ankles. Eagle feathers are placed on the head like a crown. The women sun dancers wear plain white dresses made of cloth or buckskin. The dresses are red, yellow, black, or white (tribal colors), with simple beadwork adorning them. There is no rehearsal for a Sun Dance. It is a ceremonial prayer, and like all Indian prayers, it is spontaneous.

Hunkapi: Making Relatives:

The purpose of this ceremony is to create a bond between people that is closer than a kinship tie. The ritual is for friends to adopt one another into a new relationship. The exchange or gift of a peace pipe, or a special stone, can symbolize the spiritual blood bond that occurs here.

Ishnata Awicalowan: Preparing A Girl For Womanhood:

This ritual recognized the importance of women as the source of the flowering tree of the Lakota nation. The ceremony is a source of much holiness for the women and for the entire Lakota nation. It is also known as a rite of puberty.

Tapa Wanka Yap: Throwing the Ball:

In the ceremony, a small girl stands at the center of the circle and throws a ball from the center outward to the four quarters of the universe, symbolizing that the Great Spirit is everywhere, and the ceremony *establishes* the relationship of the people to the universe, or to the Great Spirit, who is everywhere.

Humor and Coyote, The Trickster

Humor, in general, has traditionally been a key aspect of American Indian culture. Deloria (1969) points out that "the humorous side of Indian life" is lacking in American consciousness. The American Indian people are exactly opposite of the popular stereotype. They can find humor in the most dire situations. When a people can laugh at themselves and laugh at others and hold all aspects of life together without letting anybody drive them to extremes, then it seems that these people can survive (Deloria as cited in Trout, 1999). Humor is a feature of the Trickster, an important American Indian entity, often personified as the coyote. The trickster is comic in the sense that he does not reclaim idealistic ethics, but survives as a part of the natural world; he represents a spiritual balance in a comic drama, rather than the romantic elimination of human contradictions and evil. The coyote is found in many Trickster stories of California Indians, specifically the story told by the Maidu Indians, in which Coyote seems to have brought mischief into a perfect world. In fact, he brings tears and death: that is he brings uniquely human emotions and the reality of the end of life, without which there cannot be human life as we know it. Trickster stories are told to American Indian children for the purpose of teaching moral, spiritual, and religious principles. The moral and religious importance of Trickster myths and cycles cannot be ignored. It has been argued that the funny and immoral activities of the Trickster are used to teach children morality by negative example, but the most important function of the American Indian Trickster, in general, is to mediate between the human world and the divine, to call attention to the element of disorder (even death) that makes the world real and alive, and like the earth goddesses of some mythologies, to teach humans how to survive (Leeming & Page, 1998).

Application to Social Work Practice

In working with oppressed populations, empowerment practice is the most appropriate approach to take. Empowerment practice is based upon: a) egalitarian relationships with clients; b) viewing the client as an expert in her or his culture; c) valuing the client's culture; and, d) consciousness-raising and examination of external sociopolitical forces that impinge upon a client's life circumstances, while simultaneously attending to emotional and psychological issues (Cox & Parsons, 1994). To acknowledge the wisdom and sophistication of American Indian spiritual practices is to be consistent with empowerment practice.

Social workers should be informed about the world view and spiritual and healing practices of the populations they serve. Social workers need not participate in these ceremonies, but they can be supportive and accepting of these practices. Many American Indian clients are hesitant to divulge details of ceremonial practices, and it is important that the social worker not attempt to pry into secret tribal ceremonies. The confidentiality of the ceremony should be respected.

Funds can be provided to American Indian clients for participation in healing ceremonies through special agency funds designated for this purpose. This might consist of travel funds for gas, lodging, food, and transportation, if needed.

Case Examples

A typical example of grief practices among American Indians is the need to travel home to be with family at the funeral of a family member. The *give away* ceremony is as important to attend as is the funeral. If American Indian clients are not able to travel home at this time, they feel extremely sad and will usually go to any extreme to obtain the funds to travel home. They may even jeopardize their jobs or college credits in order to attend these family ceremonies (DuBray, 1999).

Another example of great dedication is participation in the annual Sun Dance, and the sacrifice the dancers make in preparation for the dance. These ceremonies are taken very seriously and have deep meaning to the participants. Many people are healed of many different diseases at these ceremonies. Furthermore, traditionally, warriors were purified before and after battle by participating in the Sweat Lodge ceremonies. After the Vietnam War, many veterans were restored and purified in Sweat Lodge ceremonies and were able to make successful transitions back into civilian life. These ceremonies have implications at the micro, mezzo, and macro levels of social work practice.

Micro, Mezzo, and Macro Levels

The vision quest is considered a very personal ceremony and applies to the individual vision seeker and his/her life path. This ceremony would be considered a *micro* activity. On the other hand, the Sun Dance is meaningful to both the individual participants and the entire community, the *micro* and *macro* levels. In the urban areas, *pow wows* are gatherings of many tribes for social, spiritual, and honoring ceremonies. *Pow wows* would, for the most part, be considered *macro* activities(DuBray, 1999). *Pow wow* dancing is not considered a true ceremonial form of dance. It is more of a social dance and is done for fun and enjoyment, so in this way, it meets the *mezzo* (or group) level. It is very different from the serious and sacred Sun Dance. People of all ages, male and female, participate in *pow wow* dances. This includes non-Indians who participate in the *Round Dance*.

Some Indian communities, such as Wounded Knee, South Dakota, have conducted community healing ceremonies to alleviate symptoms of post traumatic stress, resulting from historically oppressive events (Yellow Horse Brave Heart,1998). This will be addressed in greater detail in Chapter 10, Healing and Communities.

Summary and Conclusion

This chapter has addressed some of the ceremonies that are common to many tribes, with an emphasis on the Lakota tribe, which is the tribe of the author. In working with American Indians, it is important to research the history of the local tribes and their specific ceremonies. Each region has special ceremonies and traditions unique to the tribes living in that area. It is also important to be aware that some of the tribes have lost their languages and traditions and have adopted ceremonies being used by other large tribes.

It is also important to note that not all American Indians practice their traditional tribal religion. Many have been converted into Christianity and are active members of organized churches in their area. In this case, they would be inclined to believe in prayer and the ceremonies of their specific church as healing activities.

References

Cox, E. O., & Parsons, R. J. 1994. *Empowerment-oriented Social Work Practice with the Elderly*. Belmont, California: Brooks-Cole.

DeLoria, V.,Jr.1969. *Custer Died for Your Sins: An Indian Manifesto*. Toronto: The Macmillan Company.

DuBray, W. 2000. *Mental Health Interventions with People of Color*. Cincinnati: Thomson Learning.

DuBray, W. 1999. *Human Services and American Indians*. Cincinnati: Thomson Learning.

Fixico, D.L.1998. *The Invasion of Indian Country in the Twentieth Century*. Niwot, Colorado: University Press of Colorado.

Leeming, D. A., & Page, J. 1998. *The Mythology of Native North America*. Norman, Oklahoma: University of Oklahoma Press.

McGaa, E. 1989. *Mother Earth Spirituality*. New York: Harper Collins.

_____. 2000. "National Indian Child Welfare Association's Cultural Strengths and Challenges in Implementing A System of Care Model". *Red Voices*, ll(8), 3.

Trout, L. 1999. *Native American Literature: An Anthology*. Lincolnwood, Illinois: NTC/Contemporary Publishing Group, Inc.

Yellow Horse Brave Heart, M., & DeBruyn, L. M. 1998. "The American Indian Holocaust: Healing Historical Unresolved Grief". *American Indian and Alaska Native Mental Health Research 8* (2): 56-78.

Chapter 2

Mexican American Spirituality and Healing Practices

Wynne DuBray and Peter Navarro

Ignorance of cultural factors can result in psychiatric misdiagnosis. In addition clinicians need to be aware of the potential effects of racism, stereotypes, and personal biases that they may harbor as a result of professional training within a society that is still struggling with a history of racist and genocidal practices towards people of color and that are framed within the Western world view.

In 1996, there were approximately 18 million Mexican Americans living in the United States, with the majority living in the southwestern states of Texas, New Mexico and Arizona, and in California. A large percentage of this population has integrated Catholicism into their traditional spiritual beliefs. The church can be a stabilizing force for new immigrants coming to a strange land and struggling to survive. Those without proper documentation live in constant fear of discovery and are, tragically, ready victims for exploitation (Morganthau & Brant, 1997; Smolowe, 1997). Furthermore, coming to this country is often a traumatic experience involving economic and/or political necessity and dreams of a better life. Most of those who immigrated see Americans as people who are materialistic and who pay lip service to a Christian God.

Mexican Americans are deeply spiritual and have a passion about life that is missing in the American materialistic culture. Their spiritual soul has been nurtured in poverty and struggle. Where there has been significant contact with Europeans, the indigenous populations have suffered both physically and psychologically.

Priests and ministers have historically been the interpreters of God's will. They are seen as sacred persons and hold positions of importance in the community. The priest or minister may be the first person a Latino or Latina turns to for help or advice. Among many Mexican American women, the Virgin Mary is held as their "ideal". They value motherhood, and devoting oneself to the children is an important role for Latinas. This includes great sacrifice with high expectations for one's spiritual life. In the case of *marianismo*, women are expected to be submissive, obedient, dependent, timid, docile, sentimental, and gentle and to remain a virgin until marriage. They are also to assume responsibility for raising the children, cooking, house cleaning, and other activities that benefit their children and husband. This *marianismo* is a phenomenon based on the Catholic worship of the Virgin Mary, who is considered among this population as both a virgin and a Madonna.

The Mexican American population is diverse, and there are many levels of assimilation and/or acculturation. The religious and folk beliefs of this population are similar to African American clients (Dana, 1993b; Ho, 1992; Martinez, 1993). Furthermore, many of their healing practices have been adhered to for thousands of years and are deeply ingrained in the cultural beliefs. In addition, traditional Mexican Americans, those who are first generation, vary from those who are more assimilated into the U. S. culture. Therefore, the church plays an important role in the lives of the traditional, first generation population. If mental health problems arise, the priest may be called in to assist. The church, not the therapist, has the power to treat the problem (Ruiz, 1981). Some believe that prayers will cure a physical or mental health problem, so they will turn to their religion before turning to mental health personnel for help.

Some important concepts related to the Mexican American population that must be understood include: *curanderismo, fatalismo,* and *espiritismo.* These will be addressed in the following sections. Then a section written by Dr. Peter Navarro, based upon his experience as a Mexican American and a practitioner, will follow. Finally, before the short summary to this chapter, a section on mental health problems and a section on the application to social work practice are offered.

Curanderismo

Curanderismo is a folk healing system of beliefs practiced in Mexican American communities, which is based on the practice of healing with indigenous plants and herbs in the form of curative potions and the laying on of hands. In the United States, many Mexican American clients turn to *el curandero* (for men) or *la curandera* (for women)—these are their folk healers—to solve problems. It is important that the social worker be knowledgeable about these beliefs when conducting assessments and treatment of Mexican American clients. The social worker should not assume, however, that all Mexican clients share or are familiar with these beliefs. Many of the more acculturated Mexican American clients are comfortable with mainstream service delivery systems of care.

Fatalismo

Believing in a divine providence governing the world and that adversity cannot be controlled are examples of the traditional Mexican American's sense of *fatalismo* (Ho, 1992; Neff & Hoppe, 1993). Some Mexican Americans believe that certain forms of behavior, such as *envidia* (envy) and *mal de ojo* (evil eye), might result in physical and mental health problems in others.

Espiritismo (Spiritism or Spiritualism)

Espiritismo is an indigenous healing practice among Hispanic groups. It is a folk system for the explanation and treatment of physical, intrapsychic, and interpersonal difficulties based on a belief in the existence of an "invisible world" of disembodied spirits that interact and communicate with living, incarnated ones–these are mediums or *espiritistas* (Garrison, 1977; Harwood, 1977). The level of spiritual development attained is based on how individuals deal with the trials in their life (Canino & Canino, 1993).

Mexican American Healing

Early conquerors of America, such as Columbus and Cortez in early 1500, must have been perplexed at what they saw of the indigenous people they found, specifically those in New Spain, now known as Mexico. Among other remarkable attainments, the people all seemed to be enjoying splendid health, a bounty which had been theirs through their entire recorded history and perhaps even before. Who were these people, thought by the invading Europeans to be savages, as their civilization was ruthlessly crushed, and how does this heritage manifest in the Mexican American culture today?

The populace of the area was composed of many different Indian nations. At the time of the Spanish conquest, Mexico was controlled by the Aztecs, a vigorous indigenous people, who had expanded their rulership into a vast, sophisticated, flourishing empire, but all other native groups maintained their independence and autonomy in autosufficiency. Modern Mexico's political boundaries were non-existent–the only separations at that time being the rugged mountains, the terrain, and other natural barriers. The barriers kept indigenous groups isolated within their respective areas, so that distinguishing modalities and approaches were developed and practiced, while commonalities were still present within the various groups. Those regional differences account for many diverse beliefs and practices common to this day, for the people still maintain their respective individualities.

To the casual observer, Mexican ethnicity may be regarded as a single identifiable unit in reference to custom, philosophy, religion, dress, music, and so forth. With the introduction of modern technological advances, transportation, and communication, we do find the beginnings of a common blending into a colorful mosaic whole–a whole, however, which still miraculously remains its unique individual distinctions despite present day integration. To speak of "Ethic Mexican" as a single approach, therefore, entails erroneous generalizations without proper recognition of its diversity. The Mexican people were heir to great previous cultures, the best and finest of which the Aztec incorporated to become the dominant Indian civilization at the time the Spanish invaded their land. Mighty prehistoric Indian civilizations had flourished leaving a rich heritage of knowledge and wisdom to what is now known as the modern Republica de Los Estados Unidos Meicano or Mexico.

Although little is known of the Aztez civilization, much less is known of their predecessors and their fallen empires. Scattered records do give inklings of tremendous achievements by little- known civilizations, such as the Olmeca, Zapoteca, Maya, Totomeca, Mixteca, Tolteca, Mexica, Aztec, and others. Some two thousand years before the Spanish conquest, these Indian civilizations enjoyed accomplishments, comparable to those of Babylon, Egypt, and China, in many fields: geometry; astronomy; mathematics; and, health. This immense wealth of knowledge from preceding ages was thoroughly documented and carefully preserved in extensive archives. Tragically, most of these archives and their contents, including the great city of Tenochtitlan, were destroyed by the European conquerors.

The Aztecs had sound medical practices, using inherited medicinal knowledge, which included the use of herbs. Most of these priceless medical records of the Aztecs and their ancestors were destroyed in nightly bonfires set off by the early Spaniards. When the shock was over, and the realization of what had happened took place, then certain priests and educated Aztecs painstakingly attempted to recompile what they could. Today, the few remnants still in existence are preserved in the outstanding Archeological Museum of Mexico City.

In addition to the wholesale destruction of their heritage by the Spaniards, the indigenous people underwent constant radical changes in their long-held beliefs and customs through repeated conquests and subjugation by more powerful indigenous groups. The Aztecs were able to remain dominant for a long time, due to their highly trained warriors' discipline and to their custom of sacrificing conquered victims. These sacrifices seem to point to the emulation of higher, but misunderstood, spiritual practices, such as the ritual of The Last Supper, where the body and blood of Jesus is consumed, albeit only ceremonially. The real understanding of the sacrificial ceremonies had been lost even in those early times, although they possessed other significant, vast, and important knowledge inherited from their predecessors. The most devastating and far reaching changes of all took place when the Christian religion was imposed upon them.

All of those affected by this new forced religion found it more tolerable to add the new belief system to their current religions, rather than to adopt the new and dispense with their own well- established cultural and religious practices. Christianity, therefore, became and extension and not a replacement of what they already practiced. In the same manner, the fields of health and medicine underwent changes similar to those found in religion, although adding and adapting the new to what was already established.

Interestingly, a few regions were not greatly affected by the white European conqueror, such as the states of Oaxaca and Chiapas. Many of the local Indians do not speak Spanish to this day, and they still maintain their own languages and ways of life. Their only contact with other people is on Market Day or Sunday, when they sell their products and buy their necessities. Those adapting to the "new" religion do both market and church on the same day. There are still untapped pockets of unexplored native lore of which we are unaware.

For the most part, the imposition of "civilization" by the white European created extreme difficulties in assimilation and integration to the different cultures. The importation of new diseases brought in by foreigners, made this task even more difficult with the resultant suffering and death, which drove many indigenous groups to near extinction. With the introduction of Western conventional medicine, based upon the concept that good health is attained through maintaining a body free from germs, chaos to the point of unpredictability disrupted the practice of either approach, and adding to this confusion was the fact that indigenous people were familiar with their "types of medicine for their "types" of ailments and were totally ignorant of the new disease brought by the foreigners into their land.

More deaths resulted from these new disease (smallpox, black plague, gripe, etc.) than all of the torturings and killings by the conquerors. Since these diseases were not in the native people's repertoire of treatment, their failure to find cures for those afflictions caused devastating results. Most survivors gave up hope for either Western medicine or mystic natural healing, but a few kept tenaciously to their roots, preserving some of their original traditional native practices.

The successful maintenance of good health exemplified by the local people was dependent upon a harmonious relationship between the individual and mystical natural forces. In this, we find the spirit beliefs, the use of medicinal plants, and other natural substances to bring about positive results. The role of *spirit* is interwoven closely through most aspects of Mexican and Mexican American life today, as it has been throughout their history. In the field of health, Mexicans hold a wide belief that there are natural and unnatural sicknesses. Unnatural or supernatural sicknesses are felt to stem from the fact that a transgression has been committed through a social deviation from sacred traditional cultural norms. In some regional areas, superstitions are also part of the belief systems, deeply rooted and tied hopelessly to tradition.

Characteristically, the Mexican people have a fatalistic attitude towards death, which is typically not only accepted, but celebrated in *El Dia De Los Muertos Y Los Fieles Dijunto* (The Day of the Dead and the Faithful Dead), a celebration held in the first days of November of each year. Food, such as pastry made in the form of skeletons and effigies, is used to enhance the festivities, along with other death ceremonies.

One aspect of Mexican mythology proposes that in the beginning God created two worlds which were imperfect. Because there was no death, overpopulation soon resulted, with insufficient food for all to eat. God became aware of this great error and created a third world, along with the sun, the moon, and other natural phenomenon. As part of this creation, *He* gave everything a spirit, and by so doing, *He* made everything mortal. *He* gave each thing a predetermined time to sojourn on this planet, with no compromise about that time. According to this belief, still prevalent among some of the people, there are echelons of spirit gods and goddesses–the Sun God, the Tribe God, the Rain God, and many others. Through cosmic communication, spirits are able to assess the actions of individuals and send appropriate rewards or punishments, which may include disease and other unpleasant burdens.

While spirit gods can bless a community with the bounties of nature and healing, they can also be infuriated if they receive insufficient homage or if celebrations do not take place in accordance with established tradition. They may threaten to abandon the people or penalize them through natural disasters, such as great storms, lightening and thunder, earthquakes, floods, droughts, and so forth. Thus, it becomes prudent and mandatory to make religious observations in a timely manner with the proper offerings, such as food, copal, veelas (incense and candles), and whatever else the celebration calls for in the way of dancers, prayers, and other rituals.

In spite of all this, the spirits may still get angry and send sicknesses and epidemics. Most spirit gods participate in chastisement, which can be mild to severe fevers, headaches, diarrheas, colds, or coughs, usually of a few days' duration. Much of the natural phenomena, such as storms, overcast, clouds, and rainbows are considered symbols of and forces which spirits use to manipulate people. The spirits or gods are very important in the practice of traditional healing practices, which can be used both to punish others or for curative purposes.

There are gods delegated to different regions or areas, and these spirits are petitioned to perform certain miracles. Such petitioning requires an understanding of the spirit god one is invoking for a specific objective. For example, a traveler, who is in an unfamiliar area may become confused or sick, along with his animals, because the spirit god of the new area found him trespassing. There are rituals used to ask permission to enter a strange unfamiliar area, and if all goes well, that territorial god grants the traveler permission.

There is a plethora of gods or spirits for every need or condition, including gods of health. The gods of death can take many forms. To the Tzotziles, native to the state of Chiapas, Death is a little black man dressed in black pants, shirt, shoes, and wide hat. His clothes are dirty, and he smells of crow. Carrying a machete, he announces his presence with a whistle or by throwing rocks from the top of a mountain. He eats human flesh, that of native residents being his first choice. Although he prefers human flesh, he will also eat animals, fruit , and other food preparations sweetened with raw sugar. *Ik'Al*, the devil, is believed to live in a cave in the mountains or in a church tower (Santo Domingo in San Christobal and the church tower of Chamulas). He travels lonely roads waiting to assail a lone traveler. He hides behind obstacles and prefers to victimize and violate women. He will produce offspring of equal evilness and scatter them all over the area, thereby creating havoc. Other mythological spirits, like *Nagual*, are spirits which take the form of an animals, just as the werewolf is a man taking the form of beast. The Aztecs had a veritable pantheon of deities individually identified for their medical specialties, similar to those found in the ancient worlds of Greece, Babylon, and Egypt.

In the present day, in spite of the availability of public health assistance programs, Mexicans and Mexican Americans in general, continue to consult their own native healers, who are called *"curanderos/curanderas"* *Curanderos/Curanderas* are widely diversified in ability and in the healing modalities they employ. Some are powerful spiritual healers, some specialize in natural therapeutic processes exclusive to their own areas, and some treat with age-old traditions, using herbs and other natural source items as used by the Aztecs.

Today's *curanderos/curanderas* are neither scientific, nor as efficient as their predecessors, and are in fact much inferior for the most part. As we have already mentioned, the Spanish conquerors made it a practice to destroy all manner of records, including medical records, inevitably causing deterioration in the quality of medicine inherited by present day practitioners. However, while we mourn the loss to humanity of one of the greatest treasures the world has ever known, the secrets of perfect health, the tenets which have survived represent a tremendous wealth of knowledge regarding nature's own gifts for healing. Those who practice these authentic procedures have much to teach us.

It is generally believed that sicknesses due to natural causes react to natural treatments, while those due to supernatural causes are treated with supernatural magic-religious methods. However, in many cases both methods are used. Illnesses, which do not respond to natural treatments are attributed to supernatural causes. A high percentage of *curanderos/curanderas* utilize the techniques practiced world wide by people who live close to nature. These practitioners are referred to as *brujos* (men) or *brujas* (women), and these practitioners still flourish in rural areas where they treat the majority of illnesses. The *brujos/brujas* are descendants of the Aztec sorcerers, and they have also deteriorated in present time from the old Aztec standards, also due to the lost information. Today, the *brujos/brujas* focus upon the magic-religious aspects of healing, using ritual, charms, and incantations as they intervene with supernatural forces in creating an evil spell or effecting a cure.

Traditionally, sorcerers were not to use their powers for evil, but for a fee, you can have them work either for good or for bad. Some present day sorcerers, who are consulted will, in many instances, victimize the sick person for purposes of power, money, and control These are the quacks, deceivers, charlatans, and parasites who end up corrupting the practice, tainting those who do only good works. Some modern *curanderos/curanderas* and *brujos/brujas* find no dividing line and will practice either good or evil.

The Mexican race is composed chiefly of mixed Indian and Spanish blood; they speak Spanish, are practicing Roman Catholics, and have varying degrees of education, yet, most of the native beliefs and superstitions still survived as people continue to patronize *curanderos/curanderas* and *brujos/brujas*. A widely held belief is that the Catholic saints have united with the ancient spirits to do good deeds, while the evil spirits have united with the devil to do bad or evil works.

Since the belief in evil forces is no doubt responsible for causing many illnesses, the logical treatment for these conditions is through the *curanderos/curanderas*. Modern doctors with university medical degrees are ignorant of the treatment of these types of problems. However, those who combine functions of the ancient primitive methods with the modern medical-psychological approaches have been successful in achieving cures. Herbs and other medicinal items are used and sold throughout Mexico and Mexican American communities. Many times the very same *curanderos/curanderas* and *brujos/brujas* use and sell these natural products to the public with recipes included for their preparation and application. Some of these ingredients are very effective and useful for numerous symptoms, while others are ineffectual and useless; still others wrongly used can actually be harmful.

Curanderos/Curanderas use various methods to practice their craft. Some *curanderos/curanderas* will use what is popularly known as the *limpia,* or cleansing ritual. A chicken is passed over the body of the afflicted person, which transfers the *evil spell* to the chicken. After the passes, the chicken is killed and its blood is sprinkled over the body of the patient. Another popular cleansing is that of the *limpia de huevo,* cleansing with an egg. An egg is passed over the body of the sick person close to the skin. Afterwards the egg is broken into a glass of water and diagnosed. Depending upon the patterns formed by the egg in the water, the *limpia* can be said to have been very effective when it is seen that the egg has rotted and formed unusual patterns, verifying that the sickness has been taken out of the body of the patient. In some cases the *curandero/curandera* will extract various items from different parts of the victim's body, such as a piece of rope, seeds, wood, bones, and so forth. It is believed that, by extracting these items, a cure is effected.

Today, even enlightened, educated Mexicans consult *curanderos/curanderas* and *brujos/brujas* in great numbers, along with the general populace. Isolated Mexicans in remote areas, who still retain their cultural customs and speak their tribal language, are suspicious of modern day doctors and clinics. Even if inconvenient and impractical, they continue to adhere to their old ways, traditions, and beliefs. *Curanderos/Curanderas* rely heavily, not only upon the old beliefs of good and evil spirits, but also upon the patient's acceptance of the powers of sorcery as an absolute certainty. Contemporary viewpoints may have a tendency to dismiss the practices of the *curanderos/curanderas* as quaint superstition. Yet, just as we are discovering scientifically the validity of folk remedies, we are beginning to realize the real work underlying the healing methods of the old *curanderos/curanderas.*

A trained talented therapist or healer can do much to influence a person's mind toward regaining full health. In order to apply the principles, it is valuable to have a credible inducement, which may include, but is not limited to, a ritual involving sound, color, words, visual paraphernalia, touch, taste, or fragrances. It is actually best when all or most of the senses are used. These principles apply to the healing processes and give credence to the therapies employed. Mexican traditions honor gifted natural healers, who act as catalysts in stimulating the healing capacities in the minds and bodies of other. Remote healing, the laying on of hand, and spiritual healing are widely valued and practiced effectively by many authentically talented healers. This trust is extended to others who have acquired talents which empower the healing procedures.

For example, the public believes that doctors, because of their studies, credentials, etc., would be able to help a sick patient. However, we know that physicians are not always successful in treatments for every patient, even those with the same symptoms, in spite of double blind studies. We also know that *curanderos/curanderas, brujos/brujas*, shamans, and other healers are not always successful with their treatments either. One reason for the failure of native healings is the sorry preponderance of native practitioners, who fall into the category of quacks, deceiving the clientele who provide them a living. Fortunately, there are the rare few, who have preserved the knowledge, not only of the psychology involved, but of the many remarkable, potent, natural remedies. However, even when old traditional formulas are known and work effectively, there can be problems in their use. They are generally time consuming in their preparation, often require ingredients which are unknown or not readily available, and the directions may be so unclear that the formula is rendered ineffectual and impractical. Yet, the potential curative solutions tied up in those ancient remedies makes the efforts to unravel them of primary importance.

Principles universal to all healing agendas are equally vital in the Mexican American approaches to health. Successful studies are now being conducted by science to extract, from plants and herbs and other natural sources, the active ingredients which can be effectively used in medicinal applications. A combination of mind and natural substances seem to synergistically bring the best results.

The human body is very resilient, but today, it is under tremendous stress because of the overwhelming increases in polluting toxins in the air, water, food, etc. These toxins are cumulative in the body, impairing good health.

Only now are we becoming cognizant of this fact, which may motivate us to solve some of these problems.

In Mexican American healing approaches, as in other approaches, the simple fact of returning to the basics of good health can have surprisingly positive results. A formula of working hard, sleeping well, and eating correctly is only common sense. Allocating time for contemplation, as well are for recreation in the right proportions, has also been proven to be of great benefit as an integral part of any treatment system. In many cases, improvements from such a program are self-evident in just a few days. An important part of the traditional Mexican American lore is to be surrounded always with music whenever possible. To be healthy is to be happy, and happiness can be the best medicine. Happiness supports a strong immune system, which enables one to ward off many health complications.

Human contact is another component of good health well understood by Mexicans: having someone listen, being acknowledged, and being touched can be of paramount importance to many suffering individuals. Such emotional support has been shown to be very beneficial in the treatment of patients as an adjunct to the other therapies used. An individual's mind can even induce an unhealthy condition for the sole purpose of obtaining attention craved from another person. We are social animals; we will go to extremes to get what we need, even if it means getting sick. If a condition is in fact induced by the mind, then the mind can undo the condition in a similar manner.

The biological system, composing the physical body, has the wisdom to overcome health problems. Often, however, a disease is so overwhelming that intervention is necessary to assist the healing process, regardless of the methodology used. In most healing approaches, when properly executed, the body's own curative powers are supported, even enhanced.

Modern medicinal drug therapies are generally believed to work efficiently and fast, however, they usually adversely compromise the natural ability of the biological system to heal itself. The tendency is to rely heavily on temporary relief, modern "miracles", and a fast cure, which often mask the real cause of the problem

The application of powerful drugs with unpredictable results and side-effects can be detrimental for many individuals. Modern medical drugs can and do cause new symptoms and diseases, complicating the alternative or natural attempts used to resolve the problem. It is believed that drug traces remain in the biological system as residuals and become opportunistic, thereby creating symptoms and doing damage which shows up when other problems are present or when a low immune system has been compromised. This situation predisposes an individual treated by pharmaceutical drugs to very real potential problems in the future.

For the Mexican American, a happy new elective in Western medicine, which is surprisingly harmonious with ancient procedures, is "Complimentary" or "Alternative Medicine". Alternative approaches are giving us hopeful new answers for many diseases. These approaches explore whatever is required for the mind to induce an improvement, as well as whatever is required by the body's chemistry to respond positively to the formulations taken. The mind, by what it is told (especially by a figure of authority) and how it is influenced, can alter the chemistry in the body to bring about a positive or negative change. The smaller the conflict between the body and the mind, the more efficacious is the treatment.

In conjunction with thoughts, a negatively charged emotion can be so overwhelming that it can override the best of applied therapies. When a patient has decided that a treatment will be ineffectual, that treatment will be of little use. On the other hand, the addition of prayer, faith, confession, amendments, forgiveness, positive thinking, and so forth, play an important role in the healing of a person, regardless of his cultural or racial background. All of this had long been understood by *curanderos/curanderas* and is integral to their whole healing agenda.

Mexicans emigrating from Mexico to other parts of the world have taken with them their beliefs, customs, and traditions. In most areas, in the United States, where Mexican Americans congregate, there is a tendency to practice the old ways, including music and religion, as well as the healing modalities of their understanding. Second and third generations, however, are forsaking the beliefs of their heritage and are being assimilated into the overall culture.

Presently the most acceptable approach to Mexican American health care today incorporates traditional indigenous mystic-natural procedures, alternative healing methods, and the therapies of modern scientific medicine. Scientific approaches are readily acceptable to the populace in the treatment of common sicknesses, while for other illnesses, these great people have found a stronghold in their native practices, which they feel are more permanent and effective, even if slower to show results, and these are very much in harmony with nature.

Explanations of Mental Problems

Some Mexican Americans believe that mental problems might be determined by bad spirits or the effect of witchcraft (hexes). They believe that these problems can be resolved with the assistance of the spirits or a *curandero/curandera* (healer).

It should be noted that *brujos* (for men) or *brujas* (for women) are not used in the same way that *curanderos* (men) or *curanderas* (women) are used. In general, *brujos* or *brujas* use the power of the devil to resolve problems: *curanderos* or *curanderas* use the power of God, in a spiritual sense. It is important to keep this distinction in mind when communicating with Mexican American clients.

Application to Social Work Practice

It is important for social workers to respect the spiritual beliefs of all clients . With Mexican American clients, the Catholic church leaders will usually be aware of and involved with families in crisis. Confidentiality must always be adhered to by the social worker, however, many clients will openly involve the priest and other spiritual leaders in their situation and that is their choice to make. In addition, the client may practice *curanderismo* along with Western medicine. The client should be encouraged to inform the physician in cases of physical illness, of any herbs or supplements she/he may be taking, as on some occasions there have been drug interactions which can be fatal.

Religion should not be introduced by the social worker, but the worker should wait for the client to bring it up. Once the client begins to address his or her religion or spirituality, then personal growth and healthy family relationships can be explored. The social worker can provide support services for clients needing transportation to and from traditional practitioners, without prying into the specifics of their spiritual healing traditions and practices.

Summary and Conclusion

This chapter has explored some basic concepts and issues related to Mexican Americans' spirituality and religious practices. Social workers, who are sensitive to the part that religion and spirituality plays in the lives of this population, will be better able to help their clients resolve issues within the family, the work place, and in the community. Spirituality and religious beliefs continue to be a major factor of Mexican American identity and decision making.

References

Beckett, S. 1981. *Hierbas Para Tranquilizar Los Nervios.* Inglaterra: Mexico. S. A. Thorsons, Ediciones Distribuciones.

Canino, I. A., & Canino, G. J. 1993. Psychiatric Care of Puerto Ricans. In A. Gaw (Ed.). *Culture, Ethnicity and Mental Illness.* Washington, DC: American Psychiatric Association.

Carvajal, P. A. 1957. *Plantas Que Curan Plantas Que Matan.* Mexico City: Editorial Victoria, D. F.

Costero, C. 1988. *Uso de Plantas Medicinales.* Mexico City: Arbol Editorial, S. A. de C. V.

Dana, R. H. 1993b. *Multicultural Assessment Perspectives for Professional Psychology.* Boston: Allyn & Bacon.

Garrison, V. 1977. The Puerto Rican Syndrome. In V. Crapanzano and V. Garrison (Eds.). *Psychiatry and Spiritism: Case Studies in Spirit Possession.* New York: Wiley.

Harwood, A. 1977. *Rx: Spiritist as Needed.* New York: Wiley.

Ho, M. K. 1992. *Minority Children and Adolescents in Therapy.* Newbury Park, California: Sage.

Holland, W. R. 1963. *Medicine Maya en Los Altos de Chiapas.* Mexico City: Instituto Nacional Indigenista.

Kiev, A. 1968. *Curanderismo Mexican American Folk Psychiatry.* New York: The Free Press.

Kune. L. 1983. *La Nueva Ciencia de Curar.* Barcelona: Editores Mexicanos Unidos, S. A.

Lezaeta Perez Cotapos, R. 1983. *La Salud por la Naturaleza*. Mexico: Editorial Pax-Mexico.

Martinez, R. E. 1993. "Minority Label 'Dehumanizing'" (Letter to the editor). (August). *San Antonio Express News*, 5B.

Morganthau, T., & Brant, M. 1997. "Immigration: Cracking A Slavery Ring: How Deaf Mexicans were Smuggled into Forced Servitude". (August 4). *Newsweek*, 39.

Neff, J. A., & Hoppe, S. K. 1993. "Race/Ethnicity, Acculturation, and Psychological Distress: Fatalism and Religiosity as Cultural Resources". *Journal of Community Psychology*, 21,3-20.

Pahlow, M. 1983. *Mis Remedios Caseros*. Spain: Editorial Everest S. A.

Ruiz, R. A. 1981. Cultural and Historical Perspectives in Counseling Hispanics. In D. W. Sue (Ed.). *Counseling the Culturally Different: Theory and Practice*. (186-215). New York: John Wiley.

Schendel, G. 1968. *Medicine in Mexico From Herbs*. Austin, Texas: University of Texas Press.

Smolowe, J. 1997. "Suffering in Silence: Deaf Slaves are Set Free, but are There More". (August 4). *Time*, 33.

Vander, A. 1972. *Plantas Medicinales las Enfermedades y su Tratammiento por las Plantas*. Barcelona: Adrian Van Der Put.

Chapter 3

Asian American Spirituality and Healing Practices

Wynne DuBray and Adelle Sanders

Asian Americans make up the third largest multicultural group in United States. According to the U. S. Bureau of the Census (1996), there were 9.66 million Asian Americans in the United States. Furthermore, Asians and Hispanics are the nation's two fastest-growing minority groups, with Asians growing at 43% and Hispanics growing at 38.8% between 1990 and 1999 (*The Food Institute Report*). The majority of Asians live in urban areas in California, Texas, and Washington state..

Asians have a rich history of spiritual practices dating back for thousands of years. Asians practice a wide range of religions, including, but not limited to, Buddhism, Confucianism, Taoism, Muslim, and Christianity. In fact, Indonesia has the largest Muslim population, and both China and the Philippines have a rapidly growing Muslim population.

Asian indigenous practices include the use of herbs, acupuncture, and yoga, which all have been introduced into Western world. These are briefly discussed here, but certainly these few pages cannot give much depth of knowledge about any one practice.

Yoga

Yoga is an Eastern discipline and is considered to be a spiritual practice for the study of physical and mental control and induction of altered states of consciousness (Ballentine & Ajaya, 1981). Coming from the Hindu tradition, it is assumed that spiritual energy (prana) flows through the body and can be released from blockages through physical postures and breath practices.

There are various forms of yoga practice, which include Hatha (physical exercises), Bhakti (devotional), Karma (service or action), and Jnana (philosophical). The goal is to integrate the mind- body-spirit and to actualize "pure consciousness". To be healthy is to have an inner peace through relaxed body language, clear thinking, and freedom from fear or anger. Compassion for others usually follows.

Herbs

Most Asian communities have stores where teas, herbs, and other healing potions can be purchased. These supplements can be used to heal headaches, laryngitis, asthma, common colds, arthritis, and some forms of cancer, among many other conditions. An herbal specialist usually mixes several herbs together for specific illnesses.

A centuries-old Chinese herbal remedy is showing striking results in treating patients with advanced prostate cancer, even winning support from doctors despite a lack of federal oversight. The blend of eight herbs, used by an estimated 10,000 men and sold over the counter, appears to reduce signs of tumor growth in patients who have exhausted all conventional treatments, according to studies in two well regarded medical journals. The supplement is sold as PC SPES The two studies appeared in the *Journal of Urology* and the *Journal of Clinical Oncology* (*Sacramento Bee*, 2000). Both studies also found that the herbal remedy reduced prostate specific antigen levels in men who had received hormone therapy, a standard approach to halt advanced disease, but who were still experiencing cancer growth.

Acupuncture

Acupuncture has been used in China for thousands of years for the treatment of pain and as an anesthetic during surgery. Acupuncture is an ancient Chinese form of medicine. Acupuncture is based on the philosophy that a cycle of energy flowing through the body controls health and that pain and disease develop when there is a disturbance in the flow. To remedy this, acupuncturists insert long, thin needles at specific points along meridians, or longitudinal lines flowing through the body. Each point controls a different corresponding part of the body. Once the needles are inserted, they are rotated gently back and forth or charged with a small electric current for a short time.

Because acupuncture can control pain, it is also used as a method of anesthesia, a practice that is gaining some credence with Western anesthesiologists. No one understands exactly why acupuncture works, but some doctors have postulated that inserting the needles may alter the balance between the sympathetic and parasympathetic nervous systems.

Asian Cultural Values

Like all ethnic minority groups, Asians have specific cultures, and values deriving from these cultures, that are important to become familiar with when working with the Asian population (Mirsky, 1999; McLaughlin & Brown, 1998; Sardar, 1996; Furuto, Biswas, Chung, Murase & Ross-Sheriff, 1992). These cultural values are significant to good health, so those working with Asians must not remain unfamiliar with these values and thereby undermine this culture (Sardar, 1996). It is also important to recognize that the Asian population group is comprised of many cultures, including, but not limited to, Japanese, Chines, Korean, Filipino, Malaysian, Taiwanese, Indonesian, Asian Indians, and Southeast Asians (Cambodian, Hmong, Laotian, and Vietnamese). While there are commonalities across the Asian population, there is much more diversity among the groups, and even diversity within each subgroup (Furuto,

Biswas, Chung, Murase & Ross-Sheriff, 1992). It is therefore important for the practitioner to become familiar with the individual client that one is working with, while respecting some of the common Asian cultural values. Some common beliefs that can be attributed to the Asian population are discussed here. These include *animism, family obligation, harmony, fatalism, and saving face.*

Animism

Animism is integrated with Christianity and Buddhism among many newly arrived Southeast Asians. *Animism* is, however, a common belief across Asian cultures. The Hmong people believe spirits are part of every incident of living and dying. This involves sickness, healing, marriage, childbirth, and death. Spirit possession is believed to be the cause of sickness, and failure of the original spirit can lead to death of the individual. Catastrophes of all types are believed to be caused by evil spirits.

Shamans are very important people in the Hmong culture and can communicate with the spirits. Shamans are chosen by the spirits and can be both men and women. Other healers are herbalists, massagers, acupuncturists, and various wise men. These healers are called in to heal a variety of illnesses. The Hmong also believe that the "bad wind" or unhealthy air currents get caught inside the body, causing illness (Vang, 2001). A coin or spoon is used to scratch the affected area to restore health.

The Hmong believe that a person has three souls, which separate upon death. One soul goes to heaven, another remains in the grave, and the other becomes re-embodied. Evil spirits are exorcized from the dead before burial (Vang, 2001). A chicken or pig will be killed and eaten by guests who are not members of the deceased's family.

Family Obligation

In the Asian culture, a common value held is the importance of family (Lum, 2000). Within this population group, the individual need acquiesces to the good of the family. A great deal of responsibility is placed upon the children to respect and uphold this value. The elder family members are cared for by their sons and/or daughters (if there are no sons). This often becomes a point of struggle for new immigrants and refugees. The traditional elders cling to this value, but the children, in efforts to Americanize, resist this value (Kibria, 2000; *Vital Speeches*, 1998; Mahbubani, 1998).

Harmony

Because of the desire to keep harmony, Asians will avoid conflict (Lum, 2000). This leads to passive and submissive behaviors in an effort to comply and avoid conflict. The bases of this belief can be found in the teachings of Buddha and Confucius. This leads to the accepting of life's hardships, because one cannot change destiny.

Fatalism

A common belief among Asians is that destiny is predetermined and, therefore, out of one's control. This, too, has its bases in the teachings of Buddha and Confucius.

Saving Face

Because honor is so important to many Asian groups, saving face is an important aspect. If there is disagreement, it is important to create a situation so that the "wrong" person can save face and, thereby, retain his/her honor. This can be illustrated recently when an American spy plane was shot down over China. The two head leaders of these two countries butted heads, until a situation was reached where China could save face in taking responsibility for the plane. When working with Asians, it is important to always respect this concept of honor.

Help Seeking Behaviors

Asians are not likely to seek help from mental health services (Yamashiro & Matsuoka, 1997; Braun & Browne, 1998). This is partly because U. S. mental health systems fail to serve minorities, such as Asians, effectively (McCarthy, 2001). It also is connected to the culture and the reliance upon family for care that is needed. It is much more likely that those needing services will be cared for within their families and go undetected by the mental health systems. Adding to the complications of getting services, whether mental health services, social services, or medical care, is language barriers. Human care systems do not have adequate numbers of translators. Besides the cost of these services, lack of interpreter services is based on lack of understanding of the need that exists. Asians, who do not speak or write English, often have to rely upon others, such as their children, to interpret for them. This clouds the boundaries of the family roles and contributes to the conflict that exists between the young and the old among new immigrant and refugee families.

Application to Social Work Practice

Asian Americans underutilize medical facilities in the United States primarily because they have more confidence in their own medicine. Non Asians are also being introduced to yoga, use of herbs, and acupuncture as alternative approaches to healing the body and controlling pain.

Self determination is a basic value of the social work profession, and the client has the right to determine what if any intervention will be accepted. Social workers should respect and support Asian clients who wish to follow their own traditional approaches to healing. In life threatening situations, clients should be referred to emergency rooms and urgent care facilities, however , the client still has the right to refuse these services.

Case Examples

Case of Kim

Kim was a young Chinese college student, who recently moved to a university city known for its high air pollution and heavy pollen days due to a surplus of many varieties of trees and grasses. She developed asthma and breathing problems within a few weeks after arriving at the campus. She was encouraged to use inhalers to improve her breathing problems, but declined. She chose to consult a Chinese herbalist, who prescribed a combination of herbs for the treatment of her asthma. In a few hours after taking the herbs she was breathing better and continued to take them on a regular basis.

Case of Mary

Mary, another non-Asian student, was suffering from laryngitis and had totally lost her voice. Usually this would last for several days. A Chinese friend brought her some Chinese tea, boiled it, and strained it, and Mary drank it. Within an hour, her voice returned. Mary could not believe that she could have such fast results, as she had a history of laryngitis for several years. Needless to say she was a convert to this new treatment.

Summary and Conclusion

This chapter has addressed some of the healing practices of Asian Americans and the popularity these alternative approaches to healing are experiencing. One precaution is to research the danger of mixing these herbs with prescribed medications as sometimes this synergy can be fatal. This chapter also addressed some of the cultural values that impact the decision making of Asians. Certainly much more research needs to be done, as this chapter only begins a discussion of these. Social work practitioners and other human service workers have a responsibility to become informed about the various Asian groups, as many of our clients will be from these groups.

References

_____. 2000. "Asians and Hispanics are the Nation's two Fastest-growing Minority Groups.". (September 4). *The Food Institute Report*, 5.

Ballentine, S. R. R., & Ajaya, S. 1981. *Yoga and Psychotherapy: The Evolution of Consciousness*. Honesdale, Pennsylvania: The Himalayan International Institute of Yoga Science and Philosophy

Braun, K. L., & Browne, C. V. 1998. "Perceptions of Dementia, Caregiving and Help Seeking Among Asians and Pacific Islanders". (November). *Health and Social Work, 23*(4), 262.

Furuto, S. M., Biswas, R., Chung, D. K., Murase, K., & Ross-Sheriff, F. 1992. *Social Work Practice with Asian Americans*. Newbury Park, California: Sage Publications.

_____.1998. "In Pursuit of the Tiger: Traditions and Transitions". (July 15). *Vital Speeches, 64*(19), 605-608.

Kibria, N. 2000. "Race, Ethnic Options, and Ethnic Binds: Identity Negotiations of Second- Generation Chinese and Korean Americans". (Spring). *Sociological Perspectives, 43*(1), 77.

Lum, D. 2000. *Social Work Practice and People of Color: A Process-Stage Approach*. (Fourth Edition). Pacific Grove, California: Brooks/Cole.

Mahbubani, K. 1998. "Can Asians Think? Struggle of Asian Societies to Thrive in the Modern World While Maintaining Their Cultural Heritage". (Summer). *The National Interest, 52*, 27-36.

McCarthy, M. 2001. "U. S. Mental-health System Fails to Serve Minorities, Says U. S. Surgeon General". (September). *The Lancet, 358*(9283, 733.

McLaughlin, L. A., & Braun, K. L. 1998. "Asian and Pacific-Islander Cultural Values: Considerations for Health Care Decision Making". (May). *Health and Social Work, 23*(2), 116-127.

Mirsky, J. 1998. "Asian Values, A Fabulous Notion". (April 3). *New Statesman, 127*(4379), 26-28.

Roan, S. 2000. "Doctors: Ancient herb remedy seems to fight prostate cancer". *Los Angeles Times*, (October 21). Reprinted in *Sacramento Bee*.

Sardar, Z. 1996. "Asian Values are Human Values: Attacks by Western Pundits are Based on Ignorance, Arrogance, and Envy". (April 17). *New Statesman, 127*(4381), 26-28.

Vang, C. 2001. *The Hmong in the U.S.* Unpublished Masters Thesis. Sacramento, California: California State University, Sacramento.

Yamashiro, G., & Matsuoka, J. K. 1997. "Help-seeking Among Asian and Pacific Americans: A Multiperspective Analysis". (March). *Social Work, 42*(2), 176-187.

Chapter 4

African American Spirituality and Healing Practices

Wynne DuBray and Adelle Sanders

The African American population in 1995 was 33.6 million (U.S. Bureau of the Census, 1996). Most live in the south with smaller numbers living in the north central, northeast, and western regions of the United States. For African Americans, who practice a wide range of religions (among which are various Christian faiths and Muslim), spirituality has been a great source of resiliency and strength (Miller, 1999; Wilson & Miles, 2001). In expressing their spirituality, African Americans attend church more than others (*Jet, 2000*). However, spirituality is expressed widely among African Americans, and ways of seeking this spirituality run from conjure to Christianity (Chirean, 1997). Spirituality can be found in music (Clark, 2000), at the barbershop (Braxton, 1998), or at the storefront church (Boyd, 1998). Some African Americans practice folk medicine that has been passed from generation to generation through their oral traditions (Detmers, 1997; Cao-Romero & Bishop, 2000). Others, today, are reviving African traditions in the celebration of Kwanzaa, which is a celebration that connects those participating through shared goods and kinship (Early, 1997; Southgate, 1997; Wolf, Anderson & Schryver, 1995). Some, today, are reviving Junteenth celebrations, a celebration of the end of the lash of slavery, as an important expression of spiritual healing (Chase, 1997). Whether, the African American is a traditional, a fundamentalist, a follower of Farrakhan, a Catholic, or of another Christian faith, spirituality is important among African Americans and must be a consideration when providing human services (Jones, 1998; Marable, 1998). For African Americans, the roots of wellness run deep and have their origins in Africa (Smith, 2000).

Western Africa has influenced the world view of African Americans in the United States. There are two major themes: oneness with nature and the survival of one's people (Nobles, 1980a). There is a past and present time orientation with a focus on the unity of Earth's systems. God, the environment, spirits, and cycles of life are included in this world view. An extended kinship system is basic to this culture. Suffering and rejoicing together is common among the people with a shared collective responsibility for families and community. Today, there is a growing awareness of this connection between present day spiritual practices among African Americans and the roots of these practices in Africa, and strength can be found in this connection (Nevin, 2001;Gile, 1997).

This world view redefines "self" as an extended self, viewing community as a collective strength (Calhoun-Brown, 1998). Nancy Boyd-Franklin (1989) has emphasized the importance of understanding the strengths in this community, including the network of Black churches and other forms of social support. This is also supported by the work of Logan, Freeman, and McRoy (1990), in their social work practice model that incorporates empowerment theory and strength-based practice. For many African American elders, life is seen as a gift, and their stories show the strength and tenacity present in this group, which only comes from surviving life hardships, including poverty, racism, and oppression–an intergenerational strength has emerged, which can be used by those working with the African American population (Black, 1999).

White (1984) writes about psychological connection and interdependence, the oral tradition, creative synthesis, and fluid time perception as important values in the development of culturally relevant programs in serving African American clients. Other themes, from African American spirituality, concern issues of liberation and social justice (Frame & Williams, 1996, Morris & Robinson, 1996). These themes are found in music (gospel and rap) and in the battle for civil rights, and other social movements. Music is a form of personal expression and heavily emphasized in this population. The well-being of African Americans and their whole identity can be defined by certain important shared historical life experiences (Miville, Koonze, Darlington, & Whitlock, 2000; Levin & Taylor, 1998). Beginning with the entry on this continent of kidnaped African slaves (Bayne, 1997) through the civil rights movement to the present day struggle for economic justice, these life events have had tremendous power in molding the African American community and in defining their spirituality.

This chapter will discuss briefly the affects of slavery and the impact of the civil rights movement. Then a discussion of the African American family will offer some information for working with this community. Consideration will also be given to folk and healing practices, and finally, an application to social work will be offered. This chapter is certainly not an in depth analysis, but offers a beginning dialogue to catalyze thinking and learning about African Americans so that human service practitioners can provide more competent services to this group.

Slavery

One cannot understand the importance of spirituality within the African American community without revisiting the impact of slavery on this population with all of the horrible and dehumanizing acts of cruelty that the slave endured. During this tragic period in history, the African American survived because of his/her spiritual foundation and strength. Even today, with discrimination and racism pervasive in U. S. society, this population relies on spiritual strength to cope with daily insults and humiliations.

It was through spirituality that African Americans were able to forgive their slave masters. It is through spirituality that they find their identity and purpose in life, which is to maintain and advance their spirit of the *Divine* (Nobles, 2000). African Americans have been defined by white supremacy. Colonialism has not diminished for this population as they have been forced to give up their African American identity in order to be recognized as humans in American society. The struggle has never stopped for the African American to be able to define himself/herself. According to Nobles (2000), culture is to humans, what water is to fish. Culture is sometimes invisible and pervasive. The nature and temperature of the water directly relates to the fish.

Spirituality affects personality, intelligence, and behavior (Snowden, 2001). A strong spirit is not vulnerable to mental break down. Spirituality is the core of the being and the life force. The African American hears two voices, one Black and one White. Spirituality helps in defining his/her own identity. Spirituality has been the redemption for African Americans throughout history that has brought them through the atrocities inflicted upon them during slavery, post slavery, and even today (Forbes, 1998; Dowdy, 2000; de Jong, 2000). African Americans have found dignity through their faith and expressions of spirituality (Raboteau, Sanders, & Stevenson, 1999).

Civil Rights Movement

One cannot discuss African Americans and their spirituality without mentioning the importance of both the church and the human spirit during this momentous period of history (Calhoun-Brown, 2000). It took incredible strength and faith for Rosa Parks to take a stand one day on that bus in Alabama, thereby kicking off a social movement. It took even more faith and strength to withstand the beatings inflicted upon the marchers during this movement. The church and their faith were the rocks and mortar that formed the foundation of the civil rights movement. It is no mystery why some of the principle leaders of this movement, such as Martin Luther King, Jr., were also the spiritual guides of the soul. It was from the soul that the strength derived to carry the people forward. It was the tenacious work of the civil rights leaders and the African American community that shaped a movement that raised a consciousness of a nation about injustice, hence some justice was rendered as a result of the civil rights movement. However, today, there remains much work to do in assuring economic and educational justice.

Family Orientation

African Americans are very family oriented, and the family includes extended family, which may consist of non-biological (friends, godfather, etc.) members. The church is considered by many to be part of the extended family (Griffith, English, & Mayfield, 1980; Levin & Taylor, 1993). The church meets the political, psychological, social, and spiritual needs of most African Americans.

Church affiliation includes Baptist, Methodist, Episcopal, Jehovah's Witness, Church of God in Christ, Seventh Day Adventist, Pentecostal, Apostolic, Presbyterian, Lutheran, Episcopal, Roman Catholic, and Nation of Islam. The majority of African American clients belong to the Baptist and the African Methodist Episcopal churches (Boyd-Franklin, 1989).

Some of the ministers conduct healing ceremonies with the "Laying on of Hands", in which many report having been healed of a variety of diseases. Church services are more frequent than Sunday mornings; some churches have daily prayer meetings, and most have three or more services per week.

Social work practice needs to incorporate an understanding of the African American family functioning and a holistic perspective (Hill, 1998). Wright and Anderson (1998) argue that clinical social work practice with African American families "requires approaches that account for the clients' sociocultural and sociopolitical contexts and are responsive to their particular needs and resources. …[Social Work practice needs] a contextual model which reflects a strengths-oriented and competency-based paradigm…" (p.197).Others call for using African-centered principles in family-preservation services, focusing on the heterogenous structure of the African American families and the critical issues facing this community today (Carter, 1997). Addressing spiritual and religious issues is imperative in providing counseling services to African American clients (Constantine, Lewis, Conner & Sanchez, 2000). Social networks, such as church, family, and community, are important to the well-being of African Americans (Kim & McKenry, 1998). However, what is even more important is for practitioners to dismiss the pathological perceptions of the African American family and recognize the strengths of these families (Allen & James, 1998). It is only through shifting the paradigm that adequate services can be provided to African American families.

Folk and Traditional Healing

African Americans report having been healed of both mental and medical problems by traditional healers (Baker & Lightfoot, 1993; Wilkinson & Spurlock, 1986). In addition, herbs, teas, and other natural substances are utilized for specific health conditions. Illnesses can be the result of occult or spiritual factors (evil spirits, supernatural forces, and so forth), and traditional healers are consulted for treatment (Dana, 1993b).

Several types of healers are consulted by African Americans clients. They may be a female community elder, a spiritualist, a voodoo priest specializing in plants and herbs, and a Christian minister who has the gift of healing. Prayer groups, Bible study groups, and advice from Christian ministers are highly valued.

Newly arrived immigrants from African and island countries may bring with them their own healing ceremonies and traditions. They grew up with these ceremonies, and even though they are in a new country, these traditions are very sacred and necessary for a feeling of peace and security in a new and foreign land and culture.

Application to Social Work Practice

Adapting cognitive behavioral approaches with spirituality can help clients to overcome negative thinking. Using the client's own beliefs and emphasizing the positive features of these beliefs can provide support for clients in crises. African Americans cope with problems primarily in five ways:

1. Frustration
2. Defense mechanisms
3. Religious and spiritual interpretation
4. Acculturation
5. Problem solving

In the spiritual area, they recognize a power greater than self. This instills hope and fosters positive self-image, and churches provide group support. There are some maladaptive responses, which include the following:

1. Alienate self from their culture
2. Anti-Self, internalized racism
3. Self destructive behavior, suicide, alcohol and drug addiction
4. Organic responses, anxiety disorders, panic, depression, psychosis

The culturally competent social worker must value diversity, gain cultural knowledge, understand the dynamic of difference and the importance of the cultural self, and adapt psychological theories to the culture. The psychosocial factors must include cultural factors and the elements of the relationship between the clinician and the client. The social work profession must avoid practicing cultural malpractice.

Summary and Conclusion

This chapter has explored some basic concepts and issues related to African Americans' spirituality and religious practices. Social workers, who are sensitive to the part religion and spirituality plays in the identity and survival of this population, will be better able to assist their clients resolve issues of racism, oppression, and discrimination, as well as family issues. Spirituality and religious beliefs are of major importance in the decision making and identity of African Americans. It is now a time for healing, and this can be fostered by culturally competent social work models and an enriched understanding of the African American community (Levinson, 2000).

References

Allen, W. R., James, A. D. 1998. "Comparative Perspectives on Black Family Life: Uncommon Explorations of A Common Subject". (Spring). *Journal of Comparative Family Studies, 29*(1), 1-12.

Baker, F. J., & Lightfoot, O. B.1993. Psychiatric Care of Ethnic Elders. In A. C. Gaw (Ed.). *Culture, Ethnicity, and Mental Illness.* (517-552).Washington, DC: American Psychiatric Press.

Bayne, B. C. 1997. "Gullah Festivities: South Carolina African American Heritage-Celebration". (April-May). *American Vision, 12*(2), 45-49.

Black, H. K. 1999. "Life as Gift: Spiritual Narratives of Elderly African-American Women Living in Poverty". (Winter). *Journal of Aging Studies, 13*(40, 441

_____. "Blacks Attend Church More Than Others: Attendance Varies Across U. S.". (October). *Jet, 92*(22), 39-41.

Boyd, R. L. 1998. "The Storefront Church Ministry in African American Communities of the Urban North During the Great Migration: The Making of an Ethnic Niche". (July). *The Social Science Journal, 35*(3), 319-333.

Boyd-Franklin, N. 1989. *Black Families Therapy: A Multi Systems Approach.* New York: Guilford.

Braxton, E. K. 1998. "The View From the Barbershop: The Church and African-American Culture". (February). *America, 178*(4), 18-23.

Calhoun-Brown, A. 2000. "Upon This Rock: The Black Church, Nonviolence, and the Civil Rights Movement". (June). *PS: Political Science & Politics, 33*(2), 169.

Calhoun-Brown, A. 1998. "While Marching to Zion: Otherworldliness and Racial Empowerment in the Black Community". (September). *The Journal of Scientific Study of Religion, 37*(3), 427-440.

Cao-Romero, L., & Bishop, A. 2000. "Don't Forget Traditional Medical Care". (September 30,). *British Medical Journal, 321*(7264), 831.

Carter, S. 1997. "Using African-centered Principles in Family-preservation Services". (September- October). *Families in Society: The Journal of Contemporary Human Services, 78*(5), 531-539.

Chase, H. 1997. "Juneteenth in Texas". (June-July). *American Visions, 12*(3), 44-50.

Chirean, Y. 1997. "Conjure and Christianity in the Nineteenth Century: Religious Elements in African American Magic". (Summer). *Religion and American Culture, 7*(2)m 335-248.

Clark, M. 2000. "Letter from Abroad: The Power of Song". (December). *The Western Journal of Medicine, 173*(6), 428.

Constantine, M. G., Lewis, E. L., Conner, L. C., Sanchez, D. 2000. "Addressing Spiritual and Religious Issues in Counseling African Americans: Implications for Counselor Training and Practice". (October). *Counseling and Values, 45*(1), 28.

Dana, R. H. 1993b. *Multicultural Assessment Perspectives for Professional Psychology.* Boston: Allyn and Bacon.

de Jong, G. 2000. "'With the Aid of God and the F. S. A.': The Louisiana Farmers' Union and the African American Freedom Struggle in the New Deal Era". (Fall). *Journal of Social History,* 34(1), 105.

Detmers, W. P. 1997. "Wood Spirits: African American Folk Art Roots". (February). *School Arts,* 96(6), 24-26.

Dowdy, G. W. 2000. "The White Rose Mammy: Racial Culture and Politics in World War II". (Fall). *The Journal of Negro History,* 85(4), 308.

Early, G. 1997. "Dreaming of Black Christmas: Essay on Kwanzaa". (January). *Harper's Magazine ,* 294(1), 55-62.

Forbes, E. (1998). "'By My Own Right Arm': Redemptive Violence and the 1851 Christiana, Pennsylvania Resistence". (Summer). *The Journal of Negro History,* 83(3), 159-168.

Frame, M. W., & Williams, C. B. 1996. "Counseling African Americans: Integrating Spirituality into Therapy". *Counseling and Values, 41,* 16-28.

Gile, L. 1997. "Festival Time in Gambia: Twenty Years After 'Roots'". (June). *Black Enterprise, 27*(11), 335-336.

Griffith, E. E. H., English, T., & Mayfield, V. 1980. "Possession, Prayer, and Testimony: Therapeutic Aspects of the Wednesday Night Meeting in a Black Church". *Psychiatry,43,* 120-128.

Hill, R. B. 1998. "Understanding Black Family Functioning: A Holistic Perspective". (Spring). *Journal of Comparative Family Studies, 29*(1), 15-26.

Jones, A. 1998. "Black Catholics: Life in A 'Chilly Church'". (August). *National Catholic Reporter, 34*(36), 14-16.

Kim, H. K. & McKenry, P. C. 1998. "Social Networks and Support: A Comparison of African Americans, Asian Americans, and Hispanics". (Summer). *Journal of Comparative Family Studies, 29*(2), 313.

Levenson, J. 2000. "A Time for Healing: African Americans Now Account for the Majority of New Aids Cases, But A Crusading Harlem Pastor Believes the Black Church Can Slow the Epidemic's Spread". (July). *Mother Jones, 25*(4), 42.

Levin, J. S., & Taylor, R. J. 1998. "Panel Analyses of Religious Involvement and Well-being in African Americans: Contemporaneous vs. Longitudinal Effects". (December). *Journal of Scientific Study of Religion, 37*(4), 685.

Levin, J. S., & Taylor, R. J.1993. "Gender and Age Differences in Religiosity Among Black Americans". *The Gerontologist, 33*, 16-23.

Logan, S. M. L., Freeman, E. M., & McRoy, R. G. 1990. *Social Work Practice with Black Families: A Culturally Specific Perspective*. New York: Longman.

Marable, M. 1998. "Black Fundamentalism: Farrakhan and Conservative Black Nationalism". (April- June). *Race and Class, 39*(4), 1-23.

Miller, D. B. 1999. "Racial Socialization and Racial Identity: Can They Promote Resiliency for African American Adolescents?" (Fall). *Adolescence, 34*(135), 493.

Miville, M. L., Koonze, D., Darlington, P. & Whitlock, B. 2000. "Exploring the Relationship Between Racial/Cultural Identity and Ego Identity Among African Americans and Mexican Americans". (October). *Journal of Multicultural Counseling and Development, 28*(4), 208.

Morris, J. R. , & Robinson, D. T. l996. "Community and Christianity in the Black Church". *Counseling and Values, 41*, 59-69.

Nevin, T. 2001. "Day of Sangoma: Western, African Medicine Working Together". (January). *African Business*, 16.

Nobles, W. W. l980a. African Philosophy: Foundations for Black Psychology. In R. L. Jones (Ed.). *Black Psychology* (2nd edition) (23-36). New York: Harper & Row

Nobles, W. W. 2000. Plenary Address at the Cultural Competency Conference, Burbank, California.

Raboteau, A. J., Sanders, C., & Stevenson, Jr., R. L. 1999. "The Dignity of Faith: Lessons from Black Christianity before the Civil War". (May). *Christian History, 18*(2), 42.

Smith, P. 2000. "The Roots of Wellness". (January). *Essence, 30*(9), 86.

Snowden, L. R. 2001. "Social Embeddedness and Psychological Well-being Among African Americans and Whites". (August). *American Journal of Community Psychology, 29*(4), 519.

Southgate, M. 1997. "Do We Need Kwanzaa". (December). *Essence, 28*(8), 68-70.

White, J. L. l984. *The Psychology of Blacks: An Afro-American Perspective*. Englewood Cliffs, New Jersey: Prentice Hall.

Wilkinson, C. B., & Spurlock, J.l986. The Mental Health of Black Americans: Psychiatric Diagnosis and Treatment. In C. B. Wilkinson (Ed.), *Ethnic Psychiatry*. (13-59). New York: Plenum.

Wilson, S. M., & Miles, M. S. 2001. "Spirituality in African-American Mothers Coping with A Seriously Ill Infant". (July-September). *Journal of the Society of Pediatric Nurses, 6*(3), 116.

Wolf, J., Anderson, K., & Schryver, M. 1995. *Kwanzaa: A Celebration of African-American Heritage*. Yellow Springs, Ohio: Antioch Publishing Company.

Wright, O. L., & Anderson, Jr., J. P. 1998. "Clinical Social Work Practice with Urban African American Families". (March-April). *Families in Society: The Journal of Contemporary Human Services, 79*(2), 197.

Chapter 5

Puerto Rican Healing Practices: The Spiritual, The Religious, The Human

José L. Guadalupe and Santos Torres, Jr.

Introduction

As helping professionals, social workers are in a very real sense directly engaged in the science and art of healing in their daily endeavors. It is difficult to imagine that *what* social workers do is unrelated to *who* they are. What they are as people as well as professionals includes a physical self, but also the non-physical. Are we *physical beings* with spiritual experiences or *spiritual beings* with physical experiences? Where does the soul reside? How does spirituality and religiosity differ? Consider the expression used by many, "I am not particularly religious, but, I do see myself as spiritual"; what does this mean? Is this a statement reflecting a desire to dissociate from formal doctrinal or organized religion or an expression of substantive difference and meaning? What is the relationship of healing and belief or does such a relationship exist at all? Articles of faith, dogma, belief systems, religious rituals and rites, and spiritual healing practices are but a few of the matters to be addressed in this chapter. For some readers, even the names of the authors of this chapter may evoke thoughts, feelings, and reactions relating to the subject matter under consideration.

Within, as well as across, the great variety of human groups, spiritual and religious practices have the potential of invoking strong reaction. Diverse spiritual and religious practices are often used to cultivate and promote individual and collective strengths, to increase survival skills, to clarify visions, to sustain hopes, to glorify our essence, and to transcend human adversity. Generalizing the meaning and significance of a seemingly endless array of spiritual and religious experiences manifested among and within so many groups of people raises another dilemma; how does individual choice versus cultural influence factor into what we call spirituality and religiosity.

Language is limited by the social construction of its meaning. Spiritual or religious experiences are given meaning and shaped by "many ways of knowing", which are often cultivated through human interaction and social agreement, as well as the mystifying evolution of our human existence. As the authors move forward to explore spiritual healing practices among Puerto Ricans, readers are encouraged not to engage in stereotypical categorizations. As it has been emphasized in other contexts, stereotypes overlook uniqueness and diversity within diversity, often promoting marginalization in the name of good intention (Guadalupe, 2000; Guadalupe & Freeman, 1999). These authors are not claiming "the truth of the Puerto Rican experience", but, instead we are identifying and exploring interpretations based on personal, professional, and scholarly considerations. By the same token, readers are reminded that cultures, including those cultivated and nurtured through spiritual or religious practices, are constantly involved in the processes of becoming.

Exploration of Terminology

As a means of building a shared base of knowledge between the reader and the authors, a brief discussion of major themes being addressed in this chapter are first presented briefly. Although used interchangeably, the terms spirituality and religion carry different meanings and interpretations, which reflect various individual, group, and community perspectives often shaping experiences. The range of definitions found in the literature seems to reflect numerous viewpoints reinforced by direct experiences, as well as conceptualizations constructed to achieve a deeper understanding of these experiences. Another observation generated through a review of the literature is that the terms "spirituality" and "religion" are used interchangeably when attempts are made to articulate experiences attributed to mystical sensations occurring in the human mind and body while engaging in one's spiritual and/or religious practice. These authors agree that a relationship exists between the so called "spirituality" and "religion". However, the uniqueness of these experiences should be recognized.

Joseph (1987) viewed spirituality as "the underlying dimension of consciousness which strives for meaning, union with the universe, and with all things; it extends to the experience of the transcendent or a power beyond us" (p. 14). Canda (1990) wrote, "I conceptualize spirituality as the gestalt of the total process of human life and development, encompassing biological, mental, social, and spiritual aspects. It is not reducible to any of these components; rather, it is wholeness of what it is to be human" (p.13). Beckett and Johnson (1995) defines spirituality as "the views and behaviors that express a sense of relatedness to something greater than the self, spirituality connotes transcendence or a level of awareness that exceeds ordinary physical and spatial boundaries" (p. 1393). All these definitions seem to have a common thread–spirituality can be perceived as a phenomenon that affects and also transcends human experiences.

These authors support Faiver, Ingersoll, O'Brien, and McNally's (2001) observation:

Spirituality may be described as a deep sense of wholeness, connectedness, and openness to the infinite (or the magical, if you prefer).... We believe spirituality is an innate human quality. Not only is it our vital life force, but at the same time it is also our experience of the vital life force. Although this life force is deeply part of us, it also transcends us. It is what connects us to other people, nature, and the source of life. The experience of spirituality is greater than ourselves [interpreted as human identities / images often cultivated and maintained by the ego mind, viewed as a psyche human source that in attempting to guide human experiences often cultivates and promotes limited interpretations of that which is observed, tested, felt, touched, and sensed] and helps us transcend and embrace life situations (p. 2).

Spirituality is perceived within this context as an "innate human quality", which is not based on dogmas or doctrinal assumptions. Rather, spirituality is derived from an on-going engagement in mystical rituals and experiences that transcend mainstream models. Spirituality transcends societal rules designed to control the masses based on what is defined as "normal", "functional", "appropriate", and "sacrosanct". Rituals, such as performance of prayers, meditations, mantras, and other devices for transcending the egotistic mind and embracing the voice of spirit, act as supreme animating forces that connect the human and the divine and can assist us in attaining a level of wisdom beyond human comprehension or articulation. These assumptions are reflected in the lives of **"curanderos/as"**, those individuals from various points on the globe, including Puerto Rico, perceived as healers who have reached a level of spiritual understanding and power to heal others through touch, prayer, and an awakened essence. (The roles and function of **"curanderos/as"** within Puerto Rican communities will be discussed later in this chapter.) The term "essence" is used here to reflect the inner cosmic wisdom that exists within each of us. When embraced, our essence can guide us into our highest awareness (observation/recognition without attachment), inspire our highest potential, and direct our highest intention (awareness with attachment) and subsequent actions. Our essence transcends the notion of "good" and "evil", as this boundless wisdom embraces human experiences in terms of divine appointments that present lessons to be learned.

It is important to emphasize that although the authors are providing a definition to the experience of spirituality, the authors simultaneously recognize that even such a definition cannot capture the total mystical experience, which in its totality is indefinable and limited by language. Language, viewed as an agreed upon arrangement of symbols, is contextual by nature.

Although a connection can often be found between spirituality and religion, each of these appears to be comprised of unique attributes. Canda (1997), in defining religion, states that, "religion involves the patterning of spiritual beliefs and practices into social institutions, with community support and traditions maintained over time" (p. 173). As observed by Walsch (1997), spirituality has a personal and individualized component, while religion seems to be generally influenced by the collective versus the individual expression of faith. As emphasized in Hebrew 11.1 in the New Testament, faith "gives substance to our hopes, and makes us certain of realities we do not see." According to Yinger (1970), religion is a "social phenomenon; it is shared and takes many of most significant aspects only in the interaction of the group" (p. 43). It involves the grouping of people around a faith perspective. It is an individual phenomenon, which involves trusting in some object, event, principle, or being as a center of worship and the source of meaning in life. This phenomenon includes beliefs, myths, rites, ethos (moods and moral values of a group), world views, and system of symbols. In general, religion can be defined as a systematic set of doctrines, beliefs, values, practices, and ethical principles guiding "right" and "wrong". Religion is often based on the teachings of individuals viewed as spiritual leaders driven by influence of an extra-human authority regarded as creator or governor of the universe. In other words, spirituality can be nurtured by religion. However, it does not depend on religious institutionalized ideologies, dogmas, or doctrines. In that sense, religion can be viewed as a "… social vehicle to nurture and express spirituality" (Faiver, Ingersoll, O'Brien, & McNally, 2001, p. 2). Spirituality can be channeled through religious institutions. Religion is one of the contexts through which spirituality can be practiced.

Puerto Rican Spiritual Healing Practices–Origin and Current Effects

Many sets of spiritual and religious beliefs and values are reflected when exploring Puerto Rican spiritual healing practices. Christianity, as illustrated by Catholic and Protestant religious paradigms, various Pentecostal denominations, Mormonism/Church of Jesus Christ of Latter-day Saints, Buddhism, Hinduism, Hari Krishna, Santería/Yoruba Religion, Spiritualism, Shamanism, and Curanderismo, are among the multi-spiritual and religious perspectives embraced by Puerto Ricans. This observation illustrates a multiplicity of viewpoints embraced within a community often glued by history, traditions, beliefs and value systems, language, biological types, or a combination of these. Thus, the traditional and stereotypical notion that all or most Puerto Ricans are Catholics can no longer be perpetuated. Instead, individualization of our professional interactions, as we simultaneously engage in an exploration and confrontation of our stereotypical perceptions, are likely to injure rapport building when working with Puerto Ricans, also identified as Boricuas, seems vital.

The length of this chapter will not allow for in-depth exploration of each of the aforementioned spiritual and religious healing practices. Therefore, the authors have decided to briefly explore some of the traditional and non-traditional forms of spiritual and religious ways being embraced by communities of Puerto Ricans, in particular Christianity, and current forms of Shamanism, as well as Santería/the Yoruba Religion. The authors share some of the personal experiences encountered by them in order to illustrate some of the complexity often observed when examining spiritual and religious practices embraced by Puerto Ricans.

It cannot be overemphasized the amount of diversity that exists among Puerto Ricans, as well as among the spiritual and religious practices that they have historically embraced. Although often connected by the experience of language (i.e., Spanish) and/or by an ethnic identity (Boricuas), Puerto Ricans are a mixture of various sub-cultures, including native indigenous Arawak Indian, African, and Spanish/European civilizations. (Boricua is a term derived from the word Borinquen, further translated as "Land of Brave Lord", used by indigenous Arawak Indians, before being conquered by the Spanish crown in 1493, to define what is currently and globally known as Puerto Rico.) It seems important to emphasize that Arawak Indians were renamed by Columbus as "Taíno", further interpreted as "Peace", which was the Arawak's first word used to welcome Columbus and his crew when they arrived at the Island of Puerto Rico (Santiago, 1995).

Before the arrival of Christopher Columbus, the Arawak Indians lived in small villages called *yucayeques* led by a male or female cacique (chief) with assistance from the *bohike* (medicine man). The *bohíos* (homes made from bamboo, branches from trees, reed, grass, and mud) were built around a *batey* (plaza where the areytos, or spiritual and religious ceremonies, and games and dances were celebrated). The Arawak's religious practices were shaped by the teachings of nature spirits and ancestors, which guided decision-making, ceremonies, rituals, and day-to-day interaction/activities. Ancestors were venerated. Once dead, with the exception of the caciques or other distinguished nobles, a person's body was frequently buried under their home. After some time, the skulls and bones were cleaned and conserved in vases made out of wood or in large calabash gourds. These were then hung on the rafters of houses for protection.

As in other indigenous spiritual/religion beliefs and values, different animals were considered sacred. For instance, bats and owls, among other animals, were considered spiritual messengers able to communicate information from ancestors or other realm of spirits. Such animals were viewed as mechanisms for receiving spiritual guidance.

The closest and most current terms that can be used to generally understand such ancient spiritual healing practices, embraced by the Arawak Indians, are Shamanism and Spiritualism. Both of these practices give emphasis to the spiritual over the material. Within these practices exists the belief that good and evil spirits permeating the world can be congregated, received, and channeled by individuals (i.e., medicine man/woman, shaman, healer, spiritualist, etc.) who have reached a degree of enlightenment. Thus, such individuals serve as mediums/mediators between the spiritual and material worlds. This allows for the reception of information and guidance from both departed loved ones, as well as spiritual guides/masters.

Arawak Indians often engaged in *areytos*, ritualistic spiritual and religious ceremonies celebrated regularly for reasons such as festivity of a wedding, acknowledgment of a birth, initiations of a youth, or to welcome guests into the villages. These ceremonies often lasted several days. The use of drums (made out of hollowed tree trunks), as well as maracas and Güiros (instruments made out of gourds), were commonly used during ceremonies. Music was a mechanism used to celebrate, embrace, and channel the energy of spirit–a supreme animating force that is innate and transcends the ego mind and human flesh.

Areytos were times to collectively embrace the spirit of god Yucahú (symbolized by *cemís*– idols made from wood, clay, or stone), a time where the bohike shared the history of the village, battles fought, as well as taught spiritual values and ways of life. The areytos were also a time to give thanks to the creator and associated spirits (i.e., the spirit of the rain, wind, and the sun) for blessings experienced, such as a good growth of crops–tobacco, coffee, and sugar cane, among other food stuffs. Arawak

Indians also took this opportunity to engage in ritualistic prayers for protection from destructive spirits reflected in illness, bad crops, and physical disasters, such as hurricanes. Games were also performed during areytos, reflecting the multiple purposes of these spiritual and religious ceremonies.

Many of the Arawak Indians' ways of life continue to be reflected in the lives of many Boricuas. As mentioned earlier, the *curanderos/as* are perceived as healers or miracle workers, who perform comparable spiritual tasks as those engaged in the past by *bohikes* (medicine men/women). The term *curandero/a* derived from the term *curanderismo*, which can be defined as a spiritual art of healing that encompasses a set of indigenous medical beliefs, rituals, herbal remedies, touch, and prayer, or a combination of these, to promote individual or collective healing. Through the use of natural herbs, chants, prayers, touch, or a combination of these, *curanderos/as* perform the role of physicians, as well as spiritual leaders. It is not uncommon to see Boricuas, who honor diverse spiritual and religious practices, visiting the *curandero/a* before attending a physician. This observation briefly reflects how spiritual principles often overlap among multiplicity of religious practices, an experience that cannot be ignored when addressing spiritual ways embraced within Puerto Rican communities.

The richness of the Arawak Indian civilization and current influence in spiritual and religious practices observed among Boricuas cannot be ignored. However, current spiritual and religious ways that have also been planted and promoted by other sub-cultures, who through one or another form of migration arrived in Borinquen, must not go unrecognized. Through the Spanish crown's colonization of the Island, Arawak Indians were enslaved and often killed when resisting the establishment of new social regulations believed to be shaped and sustained by the ideal "Christian duty". Furthermore, Arawak Indians, who were receptive to the new ideals, were baptized and introduced to Christianity, specifically Catholicism. Thus, through colonization of Borinquen, new sets of spiritual and religious practices were cultivated.

The influence that Christianity, especially Catholicism, has had on Puerto Ricans has been, to put it mildly, profound. Just as the waves that brought the imposition of Borinquen's first military governorship in the late fourteen hundreds, so too they brought Spain's national religion, Catholicism. In their attempt to "Catholicize" the indigenous population through missionary efforts, the fact that no separation existed between the political and religious strengthened the Spaniard's actions. Catholicism was then rapidly and widely spread through forced colonization of the Island.

Christianity, including Catholicism and other denominations, currently plays an integral role in the lives of many Puerto Ricans living in the Island or around the world. For instance, it is not uncommon to observe groups of Puerto Ricans engaging in Catholic rituals, such as going to mass, baptism, communion, and the confessional, to mention a few. The influence of Catholicism is exemplified through institutionalized traditions celebrated by groups of Puerto Ricans. For example, annually, each major town in Puerto Rico celebrates the festivals of the patron saints (fiestas patronales).

Through colonization of Borinquen, Catholicism, as well as other spiritual and religious beliefs and value systems, were introduced to the Island. As a result of Arawak Indians' genocide by Spaniard colonists, Queen Isabella of Spain ordered the transportation of West African slaves to Borinquen, currently known as Puerto Rico. Manpower was needed to harvest the crops (Santiago, 1995). West Africans brought to Borinquen new sets of spiritual and religious practices, such as *Santería* (Gonzlez-Wippler, 1995). Since slaves were often not permitted to practice Santería, or any other of their native spiritual and religious practices, they transformed Santería to appear similar to Catholicism.

With the arrival of Santería into Borinquen, Catholic saints were blended with African mysticism. For instance, Virgin Mary or the great supernal mother's name in African is *Yoruba*. In *Santería*, the Virgin Mary is considered to possess the power of the sea and seawater, *Yemayá*. Yemayá is represented in many colors, as it is believed that she loves everyone the same. Yemayá, as well as other *orishas* (saints) such as Saint Barbara, Changó and Elegguá, among others, are believed to represent forces of the good God (Gonzlez-Wippler, 1995).

Santería, also known as the Yoruba religion, holds the belief that the realm of supreme entities/spirits, including the dead, can be directly contracted. Santería is considered to be the practice of love, faith, and magic where special spells are prepared with the purpose of ensuring protection and/or guidance. Ceremonies embraced by the practice of Santería often involve prayers, petitions, and animal sacrifices. Priests or priestesses facilitate rituals conducted for protection from harm and prepare the spells used for achievement of desired goal. While praying to the saints for favors, gifts must be presented as exchanges. It is important to emphasize that the sacrifice or gifts (i.e., killing of an animal or lighting of candles) presented in exchange for a favor are not as important as the clear intention or faith put into the ritualistic process or outcome.

One of the major beliefs of Santería is reincarnation (process through which the soul is rebirthed in another body). It is believed that one is born with a life purpose (s). If such purpose (s) is not accomplished in a lifetime, the soul must return until the lesson is learned. Santería continues to be one of the most well-known and celebrated spiritual and religious practices among Puerto Ricans.

A brief historical observation needs to be made at this point. As observed above, the roots of Puerto Ricans/Boricuas are based in a mixture of sub-cultures, which have played a significant role in current and diversified spiritual and religious healing practices embraced by this population. As Arawak Indians, West Africans, and Spaniard/European civilizations came together, interracial marriages between these culturally and socially diverse groups of people were cultivated over time, giving birth to what the United States Bureau of Census currently recognized as Puerto Ricans. This observation is made in order to assist the reader to move beyond possible stereotypical viewpoints that generate and promote marginalization of experiences encountered by Boricuas.

Spiritual and religious beliefs and value systems often influence individual, group, and/or community identity, as well as ways of life. (One's identity is reflected by an established set of cognitive, behavioral, and spiritual characteristics that distinguish one person from another and allows the assertion of individuality. Collective identity is also based on a set of characteristics; however, such attributes are shared by a group of people.) This is illustrated by the life styles of Puerto Ricans faithfully following a spiritual and religious path. For instance, it is not uncommon when visiting the home of a Santero/a, a man or woman who practices Santería, to find candles and/or incense burning by the side of sculptures symbolizing the variety of saints.

Burning candles are often an indication of a contract between the individual and the saint (s) or simply a way to express gratitude for guidance and protection. Incense burning is frequently used for cleansing the home space from "evil" or "lower energies". Santero/a also uses holy water while engaging in ritualistic activities to promote individual or space cleaning, purification, and protection. This outward manifestation of spirituality often serves as a source of strength and reminder of one's own spiritual commitment and/or practice. This observation must not be taken for granted and used loosely for categorizing individuals, as a large number of Puerto Ricans who are strictly devoted to the practice of Catholicism also engage in similar ritualistic ways. This observation supports the need for keeping an open mind when addressing Puerto Rican spiritual healing practices. Due to the blend of various sub-cultures that make up the Puerto Rican people, one often sees the richness of each of these sub-cultures reflected in an overlapping of influences within spiritual and religious practices.

It may seem elementary to note that one cannot take for granted the fact that within a single Puerto Rican family system various forms of spiritual and religious practices may be manifested. As emphasized earlier, spirituality is considered by the authors as an innate human quality. Spirituality can be influenced by one's faith community and, equally important, is the shaping influence of an individual's personal spiritual practice. As is the case in family systems within other ethnic groups, children in Puerto Rican families are often encouraged to follow the caretakers/parents' spiritual/religious beliefs and values. As it is also the case in family systems around the globe, once becoming adults, some children feel satisfied as they continue to embrace spiritual and religious paths introduced to them by their care giver/parents. Through the energy of loyalty, some feel forced to continue following their caretakers/parents' spiritual and religious beliefs. Some withdraw totally from conscious engagement in spiritual and religious practices, while others become involved in their own individual search for spiritual and religious fulfillment. The family system becomes what we refer to as a house of many rooms. Each room is part of the larger structure. Its uniqueness and contribution to the whole must not go unnoticed. Otherwise, understanding of the structure is fragmented and likely to promote marginalization, stereotypes, and disempowerment. The same analysis is applicable when exploring Puerto Ricans' spiritual healing practices as a whole.

As indirectly emphasized above, a paradox seems to exist between Puerto Rican spiritual and religious cultural influences and cultural choices. Another simple way of presenting the aforementioned paradox is by recognizing that Puerto Ricans are born into pre-existing societal norms, shaped by time, context, conditions, and paradigms. However, as Puerto Ricans, individually or collectively, continue to awaken into their essence, the vast possibilities come to the surface, providing an opportunity for the individual's highest potential to be embraced and manifested. Through this experience choices are not necessarily based on cultural influences, but, instead on cosmic energetic forces and urging for spiritual growth and evolution.

Blending of Spiritual and Religious Principles: Authors' Brief Narratives

Between the ages of five and eight, I remember going to mass periodically. North from our house, less than a mile away, a Roman Catholic convent was built when I was approximately five years old. By the age of eight, I had done my first communion with little to no understanding of its significance. I remember feeling part of a group that performed Catholic rituals (i.e., attending mass on Sunday, doing my first communion, and confessing my "sins" to the priest, etc.) not so much out of a heart's desire, but, instead out of tradition.

When I was eight, my father died, forcing my mother to work long hours outside the house and often leaving me under the care of the nuns dwelling in the convent. Living in a barrio, a term used to define a poor community often affected by poverty, drugs, and violence, my mother decided that the convent was a safer environment than what our neighborhood could offer in terms of child care. Much respect and faith was given to the nuns administrating the convent. My mother believed that the nuns were blessed by the Holy Spirit and hoped they would influence me to live a good life.

Growing up, while periodically attending Sunday mass, I also remember going with my mother to gatherings held by spiritualists and/or santeros/as. I remember my mother often speaking about messages that she was receiving through her dreams from my deceased father. Such messages were often not clear. Thus, the assistance of spiritualists and/or santeros/as was needed to enhance communication between my mother and deceased father.

My mother often spoke about the importance of protecting oneself and family from evil spirits, as well as cleansing the living space from that which was not pure. Thus, she often engaged and exposed my siblings and me to a variety of rituals that held such intention. Such rituals did not seem to be restricted to a particular religious practice. Instead, they reflected the historic influence of various spiritual and religious ways, including Catholicism, Shamanism, Spiritualism, and Santería. For instance, often at night, candles and incense were burned with the intention of expressing gratitude to the spirit guides for protecting and supporting the family and/or with the intention to pray for guidance. I remember often observing my mother holding a wooden rosary and saying a rosary in a barely audible chant. Visiting botanicas (stores where herbs, medical plants, candles, prayer books, and statues of saints are sold) was not uncommon.

As a child, I remember times when my mother entered my room and sprinkled holy water on my bed and over my clothes. On occasions before taking me to school, she dipped her finger in holy water and made a cross on my forehead. At times, when I experienced stomach or pain in any part of my body, I was taken to my great-uncle or another curandera who lived a good half of an hour away from our house. I remember being fascinated by the rituals being performed with candles, oils, and/or prayers in a non-comprehensive tone. Interesting enough, I do not ever remember speaking to my mother about the significance of her actions. The blending of spiritual/religious principles and practices, some mentioned above, did not seem uncommon when interacting with other relatives.

Once older, I have come to recognize some of the impacts generated by my childhood experiences. I find myself being nurtured by diverse spiritual practices and principles. Little by little, I have begun to understand that there is no one absolute path, but, instead "many ways of knowing" and connecting to our divine essence.

The reader is encouraged not to interpret the preceding brief narrative, regarding this author's (JLG) spiritual and religious exposure, as the totality of his experiences as a child or youth. Much physical, emotional, and cognitive pain, often promoted by poverty, violence, and addictions, was also part of the bigger picture. Devotion to a spiritual path, inclusive of principles shared by a number of religions, however, has enhanced the process of healing.

Being born into a large family originating in Puerto Rico might suggest that Catholicism would be a reasonable outcome, and in my case, such an assumption would be true (STJ). I grew up in a western suburb of Chicago, in a city with a large Latino population and a large number of Catholic churches and schools. Although I am a product of public school education, my older siblings all told me of the hardships they experienced at the hands of "stern" nuns in a neighborhood Catholic school. I, to this day, become nervous and treat with utter deference any and all women wearing anything that even remotely resembles the "habit" of those Catholic nuns from my childhood. My "Catholicism", if such is what it could be called, might better be described as my family's Catholicism. The Catholic Church, school, and baptism were all part of my early childhood, and in the case of the latter, my baptism itself came late. My mother (who had been ill, quite often to the point of hospitalization) died before I turned ten years of age. She died in a hospital (St. Joseph's), an institution staffed by nuns. My baptism, an important family event, occurred shortly thereafter and in direct response to her death. My father (who could neither read nor write), a laborer (yet creative entrepreneur) with no one to care for his nine children, raced to find all of us children suitable (devout and financially capable) god parents.

Although I have never made any serious effort to learn how so many god parents could be found so quickly, I presume that the church played a pivotal role in matching my siblings and me with those many families whose role it would be to raise us with good Catholic instruction in the event of my father's death, but I realize as well, that the "*padrino*" system is a strong cultural tradition among many Latinos. For a short time during this period, my siblings and I were sent to live with our god parents as my father worked to stabilize the family's income and living arrangements.

Another example of the influence of Catholicism, related to my early childhood, was when a grade school math teacher who doubled as my physical education instructor (an older, statuesque woman with an incredibly effective left hand style of play in *bombardment*) generously donated a white suit for me to wear for my first communion. I sometimes suspect that this may have been the result of other influences, such as *nobles oblige* (an old European phrase meaning the responsibility of nobility to care for those in their charge), but, I never actually received first communion and subsequently never wore the suit for its intended purpose. I often wonder how that event, had it taken place, might have affected my life, but, I take solace in the joy the white suit brought me since I was able to use it to great success when I played at being that great movie detective "Charlie Chan". I make this final comment to convey to the reader that although I had been baptized, and it was intended that I receive first communion in the Catholic Church, and that these are understood as important religious milestones in my family's history, I did not have a sense of their relevance at the time.

I did not then, nor, at present, view myself as being Catholic. Christmas and other holy days around that time were most often spent at a local secular organization called the Wayside Cross Rescue Mission, an urban mission operating in the city I grew up in. Here, I and most of my siblings, learned religious hymns and about prayer and the Bible by attending Sunday school. Here, we were taught about the importance of moral character and charity. As a family of very limited means, the charity was usually most generously provided to us and had come with a "rider" attached to it, such as spending Christmas in quasi-religious activities and viewing films, such as a "Christmas Carol", in order to receive donated Christmas presents. My family also benefitted from the charitable works of other religiously-based community organizations, such as the Salvation Army (turkeys at Thanksgiving) and prescription eye glasses from the fund raising activities of the Knights of Columbus and the Rotary Club.

Catholicism entered my life again in my mid-teens, when I began work at social service organizations including the Visiting Nurses Association (VNA) as a non-medical epidemiologist. The program supervisor at the VNA was a nun by the name of Sister Ruthann, who, by example, nurtured in me a life long interest in social work and self reliance and triggered for me an interest in understanding what I could about religiosity and spirituality. This influence was indirect and from what I could discern unintentional, but, nonetheless significant. During this same period in my life, I began a journey of spiritual exploration and discovery. I became intensely interested in the varied and disparate ways in which religion and spiritual matters were made manifest all around me. I was intrigued by the variety of religious institutions and traditions in the community and especially those that were attended by family, friends, and colleagues. I was also captivated by the similarities and differences one could find in the rituals and symbols of different religious and spiritual organizations or systems. Buddhism, Greek Orthodox, and the Judaic were but a few of those I investigated. I was seeking to somehow blend the best of these many traditions into a belief system that would assist me in making sense of my life and purpose in it.

I learned from my older sisters of a mysterious and intriguing form of spiritual practice that seemingly blended Christian and ancient African religions into one, practiced by people called spiritualists. These spiritualists were purported to heal with touch, tell your future, or commune with those who were deceased and even cast out a demon or two. I learned that there was a strange admixture of acceptance and denial about the nature and role of such spiritual beliefs and practices within my family, community, and culture. These spiritualists were viewed as having been imbued with special power or at least a heightened sense of awareness regarding matters of the heart and soul that was always some how beyond the understanding or ministrations of so-called medical and psychological experts. These spiritualists were said to serve either good or bad purposes. These discoveries helped me to make some sense of certain rituals I had witnessed as a child where my mother would pitch water out of a pan at our front door at midnight on New Year's Eve, symbolizing the disposal of bad luck and misfortune in preparation for a good year, or having a piece of bread and some salt stored away (not for consumption) somewhere in the house so as to insure that there would always be food in our home. While my mother did not believe in fortune tellers, and in fact referenced to the

Bible regarding the satanic nature of such beliefs, she was not averse to taking her eldest daughter to a *curandera* when she began to have suspicions that someone, with malicious intent, had cast an evil spell causing my sister to suffer unexplained illnesses. I was asked, for the first time in my life as a young adult, if I was a Christian. At that time, my answer both internally and externally was that I was not certain. I have Christian beliefs, but also Buddhist, Taoist, and Judaic beliefs, as well. In a final analysis, there is, in the writer's opinion, no overall well-rounded way of either categorizing or labeling my religious or spiritual belief system. Currently, if asked what my religious affiliation is, I sometimes say I am an "intentional faithist", that is, I believe because I choose to believe. What I believe is a mixture of what might be called many faiths, and what I practice is spiritual in nature and in intent.

The above personal narratives were presented in this chapter with the purpose to expose the reader to some of the complexities that may be observed when addressing Puerto Ricans' spiritual and religious healing practices. It is the intention of these authors to promote the idea that careful assessment and intervention must be conducted when professionally engaging with Puerto Rican clients. The spiritual and religious healing practices are only one of the multidimensional areas that need to be taken into consideration.

Working Consideration for Social Work Practitioners

Puerto Ricans are American citizens by birth, whether they are born in Puerto Rico or in the United States. Puerto Ricans make up the second largest Latino community in the United States, Mexican Americans rating first and Cuban Americans rating third. When compared to other Latino communities, Puerto Ricans have encountered the highest rate of poverty, unemployment, and households lead by single women (Roy, 1998; U.S. Bureau of the Census, 1993 & 1990). Other adversities encountered by Puerto Ricans include ethnic discrimination, teen pregnancy, school drop out issues, addictions, violence, and poor educational opportunities, as well as other forms of legal and social injustices. However, spiritual and religious practices have often played an integral role in alleviating biopsychosocial pains and discomforts.

The degree of spiritual and religious influence within Puerto Rican communities is often reflected in Spanish expressions: vaya con Dios–go with God; que sea la voluntad de Dios–let it be God's will; si Dios quiere–if God so wills; among many others. The term God must not be stereotypically interpreted, as it has many meanings for many Puerto Ricans. The term God can mean a supreme animating force providing guidance from a place called Heaven or a spark of divinity that resides in each of us. Such observation supports the need for practitioners to not take language for granted when working with Puerto Rican clients. (A client is perceived as a person, a group, a family, or a community needing, searching, or receiving professional assistance.) When an expression is used, it may be an indication that a decision has been reached. For instance, "que sea la voluntad de Dios" (let it be God's will) may be a message of surrender. Thus, practitioners need to enter in a dialogue that is based on the language of the heart and not the language of the egotistic mind.

Spiritual and religious practices, as mentioned earlier, seem to often influence beliefs and value systems, ways of life, and decision-making, as well as promote or modify behavior. This seems to be particularly the case when an active commitment is made and followed to engage in a specific spiritual and religious path. Understanding such dynamics requires more than comprehending and conversing in the language(s) spoken by Puerto Rican clients. Thus, active non-judgmental listening is important. Practitioners' cultivation of a safe and encouraging space through which Puerto Rican clients can share and examine their own narratives is not only significant, but, vital in promoting individual or collective empowerment while reducing isolation. When encouraging Puerto Rican clients to share and examine their narratives, the practitioners can simultaneously engage in a process of personal and professional self-evaluation regarding stereotypical assumptions likely to reduce the opportunity to deepen the level of trust, as well as seeing Puerto Rican clients beyond predetermined images. The practitioner can examine her/his own spiritual and religious convictions, as well as discomforts that may emerge through working within the context of spiritual and religious differences. Such steps can be useful in strengthening professional competence. The practitioner must remember that Puerto Ricans' spiritual and religious practices are often ways to deal with personal and social adversities. Spiritual and religious beliefs and practices are for many Puerto Ricans an actual experience and not just a concept. The experience cannot be categorized. It often carries huge significance and power handed down from generation to generation.

Since spiritual leaders may have been approached before a practitioner is identified and consulted, practitioners assisting Puerto Rican clients must not lose sight of their significant role, function, and responsibility. They may be perceived as replacing the role and assistance of the spiritual and religious leader. Thus, Puerto Rican clients must be approached with professional integrity through which the practitioner can recognize and embrace the relationship in terms of sacred interactions, regardless of the form of intervention (i.e., micro, meso, or macro). The practitioner is encouraged to take into consideration the varied spiritual and religious healing practices potentially embraced by Puerto Rican clients from the point of assessment to termination of services. Acceptance and awareness of where the client is at is key to effective service. Furthermore, practitioners should approach Puerto Rican clients with an opened-mind, while recognizing that spiritual and religious practices are not static, but rather constantly changing from one context to another, through time, and interpretations. Thus, embracing the wisdom of uncertainly is indispensable.

Conclusion

As observed throughout the content addressed in this chapter, although often connected, unique differences seem to exist between spirituality and religiosity. While spirituality is perceived as an innate human quality, religion is viewed in relationship to its institutionalized doctrines, ethics, norms, and dogmas. Spiritual and religious practices seem to often be a common denominator within and between groups of people, Puerto Ricans are no exception. The practitioner, however, must be alert and confront stereotypical belief systems that can injure the helping process. Those seeking, needing, and/or receiving professional interventions must not be treated exclusively in terms of what the intellect thinks it knows. Instead a level of uncertainty is useful in order to minimize marginalization of experiences as individual and/or collective narratives are encouraged, recognized, and incorporated into the helping process. The practitioner's professional competence can be enhanced through on-going cultivation of awareness generated through conscious professional self- evaluation, as well as a commitment to engage in active changes when necessary in order to transform patterns that are detrimental to self and others.

Spirituality and religious ways must be addressed in term of historical and current contexts, as such practices are constantly becoming through their non-static elements. The context, role, and function of spiritual and religious experiences must not be taken for granted in order for the practitioner to be able to distinguish cultural influence from cultural choice. As emphasized at different times through the content in this chapter, as individuals we are born into pre-existing societies and, thus, often become influenced by its norms, beliefs, values, and ways of life. However, when we awake into our essence, limitless choices are presented as well as our potential for achieving our desired goals.

Finally, this chapter has addressed some of the multidimensional spiritual and religious practices embraced by Boricuas. The reader is encouraged not to take what has been shared within this context as a tool for measuring every experience encountered by Puerto Rican clients. The authors have simply presented a piece of a larger puzzle, which its totality is in constant expansion.

Questions to Promote Further Reflection

1. What are some beliefs you hold regarding spirituality and religion?
2. How, might or might not, your personal spiritual and religious beliefs affect your behaviors and interactions with others?
3. How would you address occasions when clients do (or do not) share your ideology regarding spiritual and/or religious practice?
4. How can spirituality and/or religion be a source of strength or area of deficiency when working with the Puerto Rican client?
5. How might you continue to enhance your professional competence while serving the Boricua community at different levels of practice - micro, meso, or macro?

References

Beckett, J. O., & Johnson, H. C. 1995. Human Development. In R. L. Edwards (Ed.). *Encyclopedia of Social Work.* (19th ed., Vol. 2). Washington, DC: NASW Press.

Canda, E. R. 1997. Does Religion and Spirituality Have A Significant Place in the Core HBSE Curriculum? Yes. In M. Bloom and W.C. Klein (Eds.). *Controversial Issues in Human Behavior in the Social Environment.* (pp. 172-177, 183-184). Boston: Allyn & Bacon.

Canda, E. R. 1990. "Afterword: Spirituality Re-examined". *Spirituality and Social Work Communication, 1*(1), 13-14.

Faiver, C., Ingersoll, R. E., O'Brien, E., & McNally, C. 2001. *Explorations in Counseling and Spirituality: Philosophical, Practical, and Personal Reflections.* Belmont, California: Wadsworth/Thomson Learning.

González-Wippler, M. 1995. Yoruba–from the Santeía Experience. In R. Santiago, (Ed.). *Boricuas: Influential Puerto Rican Writings–An Anthology.* (pp. 256-267). New York: Ballantine Books.

Guadalupe, J. L, (2000). *The Challenge: Development of A Curriculum to Address Diversity Content without Perpetuating Stereotypes.* Ann Arbor, Michigan: UMI Company.

Guadalupe, J. L., & Freeman, M. 1999. "Common Human Needs in the Context of Diversity: Integrating Schools of Thought". *The Journal of Cultural Diversity. 6*(3), (Fall),85-92.

Joseph, M. V. 1987. "The Religious and Spiritual Aspects of Clinical Practice: A Neglected

Dimension of Social Work". *Social Thought 13*(1), 12-23.

Roy, D. 1998. *Strangers in a Native Land: A Labyrinthine Maze of Latino identity. Latino Attitude Survey*. [On-line document]. Available Azteca: University of Kansas.

Santiago, R. (Ed.). 1995. *Boricuas: Influential Puerto Rican Writings–An Anthology*. New York:

Ballantine Books.

U.S. Bureau of the Census. 1993. *Hispanic Americans Today*. (23-183). Washington, DC: U.S. Government Printing Office.

U.S. Bureau of the Census. 1990. *Housing Characteristics of Selected Races and Hispanic-origin Households in the United States: 1987*. (Series H121-87-1). Washington, DC: U.S. Government Printing Office.

Walsch, N.D. 1997. Conversations with God: An Uncommon Dialogue. Charlottesville, Virginia; Hampton Roads Publishing Company, Inc.

Chapter 6

Spirituality: A Journey into the Process of Self Discovery

Marietta Rubien

> The dance of life is sometimes sweet,
> But often I move with leaded feet,
> At those times what do I do?
> But keep on dancin' to see it through.

Life's journey at the moment of birth often begins with a pat on the butt. This gesture can reinforce the notion that life is tough and painful. The notion coupled with criticism, abuse, and neglect brings about an internal dialogue that is negative and self-effacing. The internal structure produces the external behavior. In other words, the quality of life is determined by the quality of the internal communication a person dialogues. There comes a point when that dialogue needs to change to effect behavioral changes. What is the ingredient that keeps a person dancing? To answer that question, we must look to people who have been dealt a tragedy and have moved on to meet life. On a recent television show, the hostess had two women as guests who experienced personal tragedy. One woman had witnessed her six year old son's death, as he was dragged, dangling from his seat belt. She had made a decision that thousands of parents make on a daily basis. She left him alone in the car, with the keys in the ignition, while she ran into a store "just for a moment" on an errand. A man entered her car and began to drive off with her son. She attempted to pull her son out of the car, but the seat belt held him fast. The man gunned the motor. She let go of her son, and he died. Another woman lost three of her six infant children after she fell asleep at the wheel of her auto for a brief second. What keeps these women dancing in their life? What surfaced was "A belief system" in *spirit* that sustained them.

A brief overview, then of this paper, begins with a working definition of the word *spirituality*, three stepping stones in the therapeutic process, and seven behavioral changes that take place. Bjorklund (1983) argues that *spirituality* has to do with the quality of our relationship to whatever or whomever is most important in our life. In other words, it is an unfolding of who we are in the context of our life. Therefore, *spirituality* is the core of our beliefs, goals, values, and priorities. It is bigger than religion, with a broader spectrum of rules and rituals. It is an awakening of who we are and that we are not alone and helpless.

The connection within each of us helps us to move from the labels and categories that culture, family, and society put on us to our true identity. We are more than our problems, our age, roles, sex, marital status, race, weight, economic measure, occupation, nationality, or social standing. When we enter the silence, and go within, we connect to a *power* that is our core, and as we connect to that core, we also connect to others. As clinicians, the inner strength to walk through the journey of the therapeutic process with our clients must come from a source that is bigger than we are. As role models, we must remain calm, serene, and connected to the person who is sharing about themselves. We must present as a caring individual, even in the light of heinous deeds. This involves the separation of the deed from the doer. Through the therapeutic process, the client and clinician get to know one another quite well. They become partners in the journey. Three stepping stones to that process are awareness, acceptance and action.

Awareness

We, as social workers, are the tenders of *hope*. An over riding question prior to each session is: "What service does this client need and want?" This question often heightens the awareness of the belief system that we carry into the therapeutic arena. Do we feel worthy to ask for what we want and need? It is through awareness that we uncover those qualities that no longer work for us. The same goes for our clients.

This chapter, then, is really about two levels– the spiritual belief system that we hold and that of our clients. Both of these belief systems interface in a session. When guided to ask specific questions tailored to each client, there is a reliance upon an "inner knower" and, whether we call it instinct, intuition, guts, or spirit, breakthroughs tend happen. Clients regain a renewed sense of hope. They become be better equipped to face their personal fire-breathing dragons. There is a connection between the client and clinician as they share an experience that moves each beyond the scope of the problem and towards a solution. The journey brings an inward change of the mind. The perception is different. The situation may remain the same externally, but internally, there is a transformation. Religion may be a framework to guide lives; spirituality is the modality to transform minds.

Take another look at the definition. Read it slowly this time. In place of whatever or whomever, insert the word "me". Is the quality of our relationship to ourselves the most important in our life? Do we make other people, substance, events, situations, or work more important? As caregivers, we often get lost in what we do, forgetting who we are. Do we believe we are precious no matter what we do? Do we believe that our clients are also precious? That belief in the preciousness of our humanness is the essence of spirituality.

Have you ever done anything in which you were less than proud of yourself, and then needed to admit the act out loud to another person? How did it feel? How did the listener react? Where in your body did you carry the feelings? Was it easy or difficult? Of course, it depends on the severity of the act, our perception, and our history. A minor incident happened in which a woman found a flask filled with alcohol at her work place. She became flustered and handed it off to a co-worker, like the flask was a "hot potato" demanding someone "do something". She was not able to do anything about it herself. Somewhere in her own history, she was stuck. What stopped her from taking the action to "do something? Why did she need to pass the flask off onto somewhere else? Was that fear? How many times during the course of a day do our clients, or us, perform activities without examination of why we did it. Perhaps the notion "behind every fear is a lack of trust in myself" has merit. This statement may present a pertinent clue to what is really going on, and what part does fear play in the therapeutic process and spirituality? Perhaps, fear can play a dual role in our lives. Fear can become a defense that blocks us from growth, or it can catapult us closer to our internal spirit, becoming a useful tool to knock down our defenses and bring about awareness.

Acceptance

The story presented in this section of the chapter was used as a teaching tool in a parenting class. The point of the rhetoric is to show that children reflect the emotions of the parents. The behavior of little people always mirrors the emotions of the caregivers around them. When children act out, parents are often looking at their "own stuff". The story goes like this:

In a land of long ago, there was a Fairy Princess. She was lovely in all ways except one. She had tantrums when she felt angry. She stumped her foot, and yelled at the top of her lungs, spewing hateful words. One day. in the height of her tantrum, she slapped her child. She screamed regrets of her child's birth and the problems this little one caused her. After the storm of her tantrum had passed, the Fairy Princess felt intense remorse and regret. She promised herself and her child that she would never behave that way again. Again and again she made the same promise, each time meaning it, but, a next time came, and the scene was replayed. She did not know where all the anger came from, only that it welled up inside her, and she was unable to stop it. Again, afterward, she felt the intense feelings of shame. Before the fits of anger, the Fairy Princess would flit from place to place sprinkling her golden, magic dust. People would often comment on how nice she was just because she was near them. When the tantrums begun, dark rays emanated from her. All around her quivered as she drew near, for fear of what was going to be said or done. In those times, a quiet hush prevailed, waiting for the onslaught. More and more, she was left alone, which only made her more angry. Her child withdrew from her and became sullen. The little one began failing in Fairy School. She was a bully to her classmates, and no one wanted to be around her. Teachers sent her from the class, due to her behavior. This made things worse at home.

One day, amid the Fairy Princess' tirade, a butterfly landed on her wand. "Be still, like me" it suggested. Princess was in no mood to be still. She shook her wand and dark rays emitted. These rays stung the butterfly's wings, and it could not fly. It fluttered to the ground, stung. A wise buffalo came next, for the animal kingdom knew of the kind heart the Fairy Princess possessed. "Stop bellowing", the buffalo commanded. Again the Princess flicked her magic wand. Again, out came dark rays that stung the tough hide of the buffalo. The buffalo had been around for a very long time. "Cantankerous Fairy, I've been where you are. I have stamped and run rough shot over others. One night, I was shown how my behavior affected others. I saw and felt the pain I was causing in my wake of tantrums. I asked for help, for I did not understand my own behavior. An eagle was sent to help me. It took me to a quiet place and whispered, 'Be still'. That only made me feel anxious and scared. "What did a tough old buffalo like me know of sitting still?' But, the eagle gave me the vision of soaring above the circumstance. It showed me how to keep my mouth clamped shut. No matter how hard I wanted to yell, I bit down. I stayed in the silence. At times, I needed to walk away because the urge to scream was so great. Pretty soon the intense feelings passed. Lizard came round and asked what I was doing. 'Nothing',I replied. Yet, in the nothing was everything." The Fairy Princess interrupted, "What's all this have to do with me?" "Move out of my way." And buffalo did so, looking sadly at her as she went off, stomping and muttering in anger. Several days later, the fairy child had a tantrum, kicking, hitting, throwing things, and yelling. When she would not stop, the Fairy Princess took hold of her child's arms and shook her, yelling, "Stop it now, or you will really get it."

The princess had learned to raise children as her mother had done. In a flash, the princess remembered the words of the buffalo, "Be still". That was the last thing she wanted to do, but, she clamped down hard on her jaw and did not utter another word. She released her daughter's arms and walked away. She sat still with her eyes closed and her jaw clamped down tight. She could hear her daughter screaming and yelling in the next room. On and on the child ranted, just like she had done in the past. Still momma stayed where she was sitting. Finally, there was silence. Momma opened her eyes and saw her child sitting close by her. The Fairy Princess scooped her child in her arms and called to the old buffalo. The old buffalo came. "In the silence, I heard my child's pain. In the silence, I felt my own. In unison, the buffalo, the butterfly, and the eagle whispered in the Fairy Princess' ear, the secret to peace is "Be still". "I'll remember", she whispered back, and she did.

Where in the story is the real intervention? What was the real crisis? How many times had the momma made a deal with herself and her child? How many times did that deal get broken? How will the Fairy Princess remember new behavior the next time those intense feelings surface and old behaviors come to stalk? Is the real intervention a spiritual one? For a change to take place there needs to be a shift in the mental process and that takes place on an internal level.

Action

There is a thought, a notion that states: "Faith the size of a mustard seed" will get you through. An action step then may be to "Keep on dancing" forward in spite of the feelings of resistance. A tool that can be utilized as a visual for clients in those trying times is a can of mustard seeds. The seeds become a reminder of how little faith is needed. Faith in them tenders hopes and produces options. Clients often feel stuck in their lives. They are floundering with life on life's terms. "Feeling stuck" often produces a clinical depression. Adding a substance (alcohol, illegal drugs, sugar, and cigarettes) often compounds that depression. Parents, under the influence, have made choices that place children in unsafe environments. Substance abuse has been called the "robber of the soul". How does the clinician, who is floundering with her/his own spirituality, interface with a client who has lost hope?

What form of support can we, as clinicians, give those clients that have experienced devastating life events through no fault of their own, such as their child being diagnosed with a life threatening illness? Where do people receive the courage to change their lives or get on with the business of living? We, who are the role models, called clinicians, often reveal to our clients their innate goodness. Many, for the first, time learn the freedom of choice. This freedom of choice is best depicted in a story about a famous ballet dancer, Rudolf Nureyev, who defected from Russia to the West on May 11,1961. He decided to seize the opportunity of the moment. He chose to defect. He had flown from Leningrad to dance in Paris. He left everything behind and placed himself in the hands of the French police. He did not know his future; he only knew he could not go back to where he came from. How many of our clients face that same dilemma? In the moment of defection, Nureyev took courage and decided to shape his destiny. He took action.

Often, with our clients, we face the passiveness of wanting to change, but like the woman with the flask they want others "do it for them". Someone else can make the choice, because the risk seems so insurmountable. The fear of making a mistake or making the wrong decision may keep us stuck. Where does the courage to propel us into action come from? What or whom breaks through the human paradox of seeing our own creative abilities and choosing to do something about it for our selves. Nureyev prayed for freedom. He wanted what most of us want for ourselves, self- determination. For Nureyev, dancing is freedom. He knew what he wanted and that was his miracle, but he needed to want it enough to risk everything for it. That was his spiritual journey.

People addicted to a substance often risk everything for their "fix", but would you call that a spiritual journey? I think not, for on such a journey, there are principles that lend themselves to an improved quality of relationship to whatever or whomever is important. Often the destruction of the addiction leads to the Twelve-Step Program of Alcoholics Anonymous. This program is based on spiritual principles of love (awareness), forgiveness (acceptance), and trust (action), but what does that mean in every day language. For the recovering alcoholic, it means *to admit: 1) powerlessness; 2) surrender to a Power (Spirit) greater than self; and, 3) to take a simple action: not take the first drink.* By the admission, surrender, and action process, one day at a time, there is a reprieve from drinking alcohol, but, what is the ingredient that brings the alcoholic to the brink of change? Many believe it is the *spirit of grace*.

The founder of Alcoholics Anonymous was a man whose life was governed by the next drink. He had "sworn off" many times. Alcohol had a grip, and he would return to it. This would cause him to be institutionalized for the insane. He posed a danger to himself. Many often died of alcohol. In those days, he had done the usual things and was pronounced "incurable" by the learned at the time. The only course, "treatment", was institutionalization for the insane. It was thought that the disease of alcoholism was a moral issue, not enough will power. A revolutionary notion was to admit defeat and surrender to a Power greater than alcohol one day at a time, but in the surrender process, a course of action was laid out to remain sober. Action in the form of service to others was the ticket. An experience of a connection with his Creator led him to write a chapter in what is now known to the fellowship as the "Big Book" of Alcoholics Anonymous. In this chapter, he outlines a spiritual life by utilizing twelve simple steps. He states they are simple, but not easy. In living these 12-steps, there is a reprieve from the disease of alcoholism, but what was the connection to the Creator that led Bill Wilson to write the chapter for a sober life when all around him were dying of the disease? What is it in all of us that we experience an epiphany at crucial times in our lives, and our lives are never the same again. The nugget is spiritual in nature, for left to our own devices, we would continue on our merry way of destruction. People who are addicted to substances or compulsive behaviors need a powerful internal ally to catapult them from the life style they are living into a new dimension. Who or what causes the shift in consciousness?

What one ingredient keeps people from "slipping back" and gives them the strength to make changes in their life? The Big Books (Alcoholics Anonymous and the Bible) suggest a belief in a "Power Bigger than we are". The Big Book of AA suggests twelve steps that lead towards a spiritual life. These are the following:

1. We admitted we were powerless over alcohol-that lives are unmanageable.
2. Came to believe that a Power greater than ourselves could restore us to sanity.

3. Made a decision to turn our will and our lives over to the care of God, *as we understood Him.*

4. Made a searching and fearless moral inventory of ourselves.

5. Admitted to God, to ourselves, and to another human being the exact nature of our wrongs.

6. Were entirely ready to have God remove all these defects of character.

7. Humble asked Him to remove our shortcomings.

8. Made a list of all persons we had harmed, and became willing to make amends to them all.

9. Made direct amends to such people wherever possible, except when to do so would injure them or others.

10. Continued to take personal inventory and when we were wrong promptly admitted it.

11. Sought through prayer and meditation to improve our conscious contact with God, *as we understood Him,* praying only for knowledge of His will for us and the power to carry that out.

12. Having had a spiritual awakening as the result of these steps, we tried to carry this message to alcoholics, and to practice these principles in all our affairs.

The steps suggest a course of life, a handbook if you will, which include admission of defeat, surrender, letting go, guidance, and taking action. So what does this all have to do with social work? Social work is the establishing of rapport with our clients, a connection between one individual and another. This rapport, I call the heart connection. This heart connection enables the client to share and work through the "tough stuff" in their lives, because that individual is heard and accepted.

Acceptance becomes most crucial in the process of facing self, moving from the false idea of being bad or helpless. and moving into the realm of healing. Shame and guilt stems from false ideas. The universal longing in all of us is to be seen and heard for who we really are, not for what we have done. It is usually our deeds that need to be changed, because the acts have caused pain either to others or us.

Yet clients come to us with feelings of shame, guilt, anger, and remorse that seem to engulf and overwhelm them. They come to us full of fear and that fear plays out in a variety of ways: defended; resistive; argumentative; sad; anxious; and, withdrawn. Underneath any of these feelings, the vulnerable self is yelling "see me, know me". There once was a man who came into the agency with a case history that included domestic violence, substance abuse, and a jail sentence. He sat in the office and wept, because his history was what the judge had seen, and he was deprived seeing his children. He desperately wanted to see them, for it appeared he loved them very much. He stated, "I know you read all about my past and that is coloring how you are acting towards me. Please see me! The *me* sitting here in this chair and talking to you in this minute." I asked him to describe himself to me. He had a list of attributes that was different than the printed word said about him. His list included, "I'm kind to my children, I work hard to support my family, I do wood working with my hands, I laugh and cry, and I cook grommet meals and play baseball." "Does that paper say any of that?"

A simple request was by this man, "Teach me about you. Help me see the real you." Of course, there were behavioral changes he needed to make, but in order for any of those changes to take place, a joining with him in his vision of himself, both positive and negative, needed to take place. The negative self-image is more readily shared in an atmosphere of acceptance. When individuals and families begin the session with a prayer or moment of connection with their belief system, they move through the therapeutic arena faster than those who do not. Defenses were more readily dropped, and hearts opened into compassion. Being seen, heard, and accepted seems to be a recurrent theme in sessions.

Behavioral changes take place when we become aware of the negative impact old behaviors have had, accept the doer as human and bigger than the deed, and then take a course of action that brings a sense of empowerment. Our clients teach us about themselves. When asked, "What gets you up in the morning?", many reply, "I just know that things will get better." Is that a statement of faith? One of spirituality? Are they interchangeable? What is the indefinable ingredient that causes motivation in clients? Is it only pain? Why does pain propel some clients to move toward action and some clients stay "stuck"? Is it the connection to *spirit*? Are we, as clinicians, the conduit to that *spirit*? We are lenders of hope in trying times. We lend a vision of what could be, asking our clients to "see it with us". What are we seeing, and who or what conveys that vision to us?

In our own trying times, where do we go for our own connection to the "Power bigger than we are?" Most of the time, it is a movement toward inside of us. In the quiet, we are "gathered" or quieted. What causes the quiet? When there is a shift from the outer world to the inner one, how does it apply to the clinical aspect of social work? We, both our clients and ourselves, are multidimensional beings. We suit up and show up in our lives on a daily basis. We are more than our problems, our jobs, our roles, and our material trappings, our worries, or our anxieties. At the point that we, as clinicians, interface with our clients, we have our mental and emotional suitcases packed with "stuff" that "colors our perceptions" to the situation at hand. We need to keep our own suitcases clear as we help unpack our clients suitcases. Who or what helps us to look at each of the items, as they are uncovered. Our job is to hold up the items that may cause pain in our clients and hold steady to the vision that these items may need to be discarded, altered, or laundered, but who helps us to hold steady during these times when our clients are still attached to the items and are resistant to either show us or discard them. How do we "keep the faith" day after day? How do we "lend the vision" to a client who is bogged down in dirty clothes or useless items in the suitcase? How do we keep from mixing our baggage with theirs? The answer for me is spirituality. We all have a core need: to be accepted for whom we are. When we get the idea, WE CAN

ACCEPT OURSELVES, just like we are in the moment, warts, wrinkles, and behaviors, then we move into the realm of spirit. We move from judgement into awareness. Awareness brings change. Awareness is a "Spiritual Awakening", and we enter the realm of possibilities. Then we change our minds. That change brings a different course of action. I have a cartoon in my office that depicts a big dragon standing over a person covered with smoke. The caption states, "Sometimes the dragon wins." How true! But, what does it take to get up? Because lying on the ground toasted keeps us stuck. "Ain't it awful" statements compounds the situation. Yes, it is. Now what? The getting up is the part of life that asks us to move into spirit, into hope. Do we have the courage to face the dragon again? Even after being toasted? Sometimes, we stand before the dragon, quaking, with what looks like a small water gun. The action it took to stand up is the miracle, because there was a change. We learned, and we survived. We must give ourselves and each other credit for the courage. We must renew our spirit daily, so that we may lend hope to those who are lost.

A little boy's behavior was enough to drive his parents into a frenzied state. His family was in despair and was at a breaking point of needing a respite. They were torn between the love they had for him and coping with his offensive behavior every single day. They were worn out, and the "ideal" solution was to send him away. So, both the little boy and his family played the game "come close, but don't you dare". They would connect with a hug or a gentle pat for a few seconds and then threat "if you don't behave, I'll send you away". His negative behavior accelerated. The cycle repeats itself several times a day, day in and day out. This little boy asked at one point in therapy, "Can I have more than one chance to be good?" He went on to state, "I am bad, and this makes me do bad things." Who needs to change in this family system and how? As clinicians, we can look in our "bag of tricks" with suggestions for behavioral modification and parenting techniques. We can make appropriate referrals for medication for the little boy's mood and impulse, and we can monitor changes.

However, on what level is the real work being done? Who is doing it? What makes some clients embrace the internal work that needs to be done and others stay in denial? Often it is their spiritual awakening.

An incident will be the catalysis to propel clients to seek therapy. They come in wanting to be fixed or have someone fixed who is causing them stress. They feel helpless, hopeless, depressed, and stuck. They come looking for an external something that will "make it all better". Many are hopeless of having things ever change, and then become angry when they realize "Change is an inside job." Many leave therapy at this point, "because it is too hard". Those who stay in the milieu, begin to explore their internal landscape. Often belief in a concept of a god comes into question. When the belief system centers on a punishing, critical authority figure, who is out to "get them", the internal dialogue mirrors that belief. When the issued is explored, childhood beliefs are brought to the forefront. After all, their first god was a parent. How that care was administered formulated a sense of self, bad or good. Then there was the aspect of religion. Was god a punishing, judgmental one that enhanced their parents' view of them? These questions often become a spiritual journey to change the sense of self. We, as clinicians, walk with our clients in that journey, and we often hear their cry. Many of us have heaved the same cry. We lend an ear. We lend support. We take their hand, and we walk together, exploring those aspects of self that have caused pain and those that have caused joy. We voice and question beliefs that are no longer valid; for example, "I am bad and do bad things, I am unworthy of being loved, or I am such a mess." This internal belief about self produces external behaviors that can produce abuse. In that case, in spite of a spiritual connection with clients, social workers are mandated reporters. Reporting suspected abuse usually brings a rupture in the therapeutic process. The internal conflict we feel many times is mirrored in the angry response of the reported client. Sometimes, we can move past the report. If the abuse is substantiated, dire consequences result regarding custody of children. So both internal and external changes must be made in order to insure safety.

The spiritual journey is the change process. Clients who make the internal shifts exhibit seven identified behavioral changes. These are as follows:

1. A revised belief system
2. Renewed energy
3. Passion for or purpose in life
4. A strategy or plan for their life
5. Clarity of values
6. Ability to bond and establish healthy rapport with self and others
7. Mastery of both internal and external communication

An illustration of these behavioral changes is best illustrated in the next case history.

In the process of adopting a severely disabled little boy, a single mom's application was denied. This woman had grown to love this little boy, since they had a history since birth. She felt devastated. She yelled and shared her frustration and sadness. She went into the silence for a few days and then began to take action. For her the word "no" did not take on the conation of rejection, wrong, or bad. She revised her belief system, and with renewed energy, she took it to mean a "bigger yes". Her passion or purpose in life was to bring the little boy "home". She told me of her plan. She was moving closer to where he lived (at that time, he was placed out of state in a group home), so she could be "up close and personal". She was willing to start the process all over again, because "there is a hole in my family. Just because a family member is no longer with you is not a reason to give up and forget that member." She was able to master the "ain't it awful" dialogue in her head and transform it into options. She went inside and drew on her courage and the integrity of whom she was and what she wanted to do, but first, she went into the silence.

We are taught, as clinicians, that silence is an important part of the therapeutic process for us, as well as our clients. Often times, we are uncomfortable in the silence, but, in the mind chatter or noise of everyday life, how can we pay attention to the spirit (still small voice) within? We teach the active art of listening by staying still and just being present with our clients. An example of the gift of silence was brought home through a friend.

This writer was moaning and gnashing her teeth about a situation that shook an accustomed belief system. This friend had experienced a similar situation and knew there were no answers. Going through the situation and feeling the gamut of emotions was the only course of action needed to be taken. Quietly and gently, she reached out her hand. That simple gesture in silence was a heart connection. There is space in the silence for tears to break open the hopeless, helpless feelings. It takes strength to sit in the silence and attend "suffering". It is in the silence that we connect with our spirit. It is in the silence that our truth is registered in our hearts. It is in the loving gift of silence that we can connect with one another. As clinicians, we must go into our own silent world through prayer, meditation, walking, and sitting quietly. We must become comfortable with the silence, before we can walk through it with our clients. For it is there that our essence and spirit resides. William Shakespeare is quoted with stating: "Go to your bosom: Knock there, and ask your heart what it doth know." So how do we teach our clients how to sit in the silence?

The demonstration of active silent listening during a session or two conveys this wonderful tool. Moving from the arena of "fixing" into the realm of our own spiritual connection with our clients and ourselves is central in the helping relationship.

What do we each need from one another? Validation that we are precious! Acceptance of our humanness! A way of living, a guide book if you will, that is spiritual in nature; the twelve steps of Alcoholics Anonymous is but one path. Often therapy takes on a spiritual nature because the quality of our relationship with whatever or whoever is important in our life is improved. In short, we want a miracle. Usually the miracle comes in the form of strength to take a course of action that changes our lives.

What of our employers, the agencies that we work for? Do they foster spirituality in our clients or us? How do we incorporate our spirituality in the workplace? As catalysts for change, the social worker interfaces with resistance and then must deal with that resistance on the meso, as well as the micro level. The constant friction can erode our values. We can become battle weary and burned out. So, we must turn within and feel the nurturance of our own Spiritual Journey. "Social Work is not for wimps!"

In every spiritual journey, there are miracles. They can be as inconspicuous as a change of mind, or out right obvious. The following story illustrates a child's faith and a miracle. It became an instrument to support a course of action that produced an internal shift in her and those she touched:

The Miracle: A True Story
(author unknown)

Tess was a precious eight year old, when she heard her mom and dad talking about her little brother, Andrew. All she knew was that he was very sick, and they were completely out of money. They were moving to an apartment complex next month because Daddy didn't have the money for the doctor bills and our house. Only a very costly surgery could save him now, and it was looking like there was no one to loan them the money. She heard Daddy say to her tearful Mother with whispered desperation, "Only a miracle can save him now."

Tess went to her bedroom and pulled a glass jelly jar from its hiding place in the closet. She poured all the change out on the floor and counted it carefully–three times, even. No chance here for mistakes. Carefully placing the coins back in the jar and twisting on the cap, she slipped out the back door and made her way six blocks to Rexall's Drug Store with the big Indian Chief sign above the door. She waited patiently for the pharmacist to give her some attention, but he was too busy at this moment. Tess twisted her feet to make a scuffing noise. Nothing! She cleared her throat with the most disgusting sound she could muster. No good! Finally, she took a quarter from her jar and banged it on the glass counter. That did it!

"And what do you want?" the pharmacist asked in an annoyed tone of voice. "I'm talking to my brother from Chicago whom I haven't seen in ages," he said without waiting for a reply to his question.

"Well, I want to talk to you about my brother," Tess answered back in the same annoyed tone. "He's really, really sick... and I want to buy a miracle."

"I beg your pardon?" said the pharmacist.

"His name is Andrew, and he has something bad growing inside his head, and my Daddy says only a miracle can save him now. So how much does a miracle cost?"

"We don't sell miracles here, little girl. I'm sorry but I can't help you," the pharmacist said, softening a little.

"Listen, I have the money to pay for it. If it isn't enough, I will get the rest. Just tell me how much it costs."

The pharmacist's brother was a well-dressed man. He stooped down and asked the little girl, "What kid of miracle does your brother need?"

"I don't know," Tess replied with her eyes welling up. "I just know he's really sick, and Mommy says he needs an operation. But my Daddy can't pay for it, so I want to use my money.

"How much do you have?" asked the man from Chicago.

"One dollar and eleven cents," Tess answered barely audibly. "And it's all the money I have, but I can get some more if I need too."

"Well, what a coincidence," smiled the man. "A dollar and eleven cents—-the exact price of a miracle for little brothers." He took her money in one hand, and with the other hand he grasped her mitten and said, "Take me to where you live. I want to see your brother and meet your parents. Let's see if I have the kind of miracle you need."

That well dressed man was Dr. Carlton Armstrong, a surgeon, specializing in neuro-surgery. The operation was completed without charge, and it wasn't long until Andrew was home again and doing well. Mom and Dad were happily talking about the chain of events that had led them to this place.

"That surgery," her mother whispered, "was a real miracle. I wonder how much it would have cost?"

Tess smiled. She knew exactly how much a miracle cost... one dollar and eleven cents...plus the faith of a little child.

A miracle is not the suspension of natural law, but the operation of a higher law...

References

Alcoholic Anonymous. 1976. *Alcoholics Anonymous* (third edition). New York: Alcoholics Anonymous World Services, Inc.

Bjorklund, P. *1983. What is Spirituality?* New York: Hazelden Foundation.

Chapter 7

Spiritually Rooted Social Work

Sarah Rose

Social work is an extraordinary undertaking. Social workers make themselves available to address every type of human problem that exists. The range of human problems and sufferings facing our world in the year 2001 are expansive and complex, including: dramatic increases in poverty and economic disparity throughout the world; staggering rates of population growth; an alarming amount of environmental degradation; and, a prevalence of violence. In America, domestic violence, substance abuse, racism, homelessness, an ever-growing prison population, violence in schools, and numerous other problems affect our lives. In the context of all of these social dilemmas, the social worker chooses a career of social service.

The inherent uncertainty of life itself underlies all of the problems mentioned above. Universal passages and transitions challenge us throughout our lives and culminate in our final passage of death. Problems, passages, and transitions break down our assumptions, revealing to us our "not knowing" in the face of deeper, transpersonal meaning. Such experiences challenge us to the very core and have the power to catalyze extraordinary metamorphoses as our understanding deepens.

Essential to the integrity of our social work practice is our honesty in the face of our own humanness. All human beings experience life challenges and passages, including helping professionals, such as social workers.

Furthermore, social workers must actively address our own process of transformation as we endeavor to assist others, and we are only able to learn, grow, and mature if we have the courage to admit what we do not know. Reaching into the unknown opens us to hidden resources.

Social workers assist clients and client systems, that are debilitated due to the suffering of woundedness and upheaval. Debilitation implies a state of partial or complete powerlessness in the face of overwhelming negative circumstance. However, suffering becomes a catalyst for transformation and healing when the "victims" find a way to reach beyond their perceived limitations and habitual perspectives to access resources that sustain and empower them.

McNiff (1992) states that pathology and wounds open us to the life of the soul. This opening takes place only when one's rigidity or self-control is lost or relinquished, at which point, there is an opening to ultimate truths that were previously unknown. According to Ornish (1997), "Suffering in any of its many forms, can be a doorway for real transformation, beyond just physical and behavioral changes" (p. 14). Discomfort pushes individuals past their perceived limits, accessing resources they were previously unaware of (Chodron, 1997; McNiff, 1992). There is meaning in every moment; for example, pain has many implications. It is wise to open our hearts and minds to the message behind the pain in order to understand its cause, rather than merely taking a pain killer (Chodron, 1997; Ornish, 1997). This is where the healing process towards wholeness and awareness begins. Concentration camp survivor, Victor Frankle, said "Man is willing to shoulder suffering as soon and as long as he can see meaning in it" (The Dalai Lama & Cutler, 1998, p. 199).

Spirituality

Vaughan (1991) wrote: "The spiritual journey does lead us from fear to love, from ignorance to understanding, and from bondage to freedom" (p.

118). Spirituality is infinite and all pervasive, truly beyond conceptualization, surpassing any dogma. As soon as one begins to describes spirituality in words, one conceptualizes and objectifies it (Tolliver, 1997; Sermabeikian, 1994; Moore, 1992). As Kurtz and Ketchum (1992) so aptly put it: "When we attempt to 'define' spirituality, we discover not its limits, but our own" (p. 14). Coweley and Derezotes (1994) explain spirituality as being "subjective, transrational, non-local and non-temporal" (p. 32). This is why there are major spiritual traditions which avoid naming it. For example, the Jewish people do not pronounce the Hebrew name for "God", and Buddhists use general terms like "suchness", "emptiness", and "primordial wisdom nature". Spirituality has been referred to simply as *truth* or that which is *real* (Remen, 1996; Watson, 1994). Jung found spirituality to be the essence of our human nature (Sermabeikian, 1994). Derezotes points out that the term "spirit" has been associated with breath and defined literally as the essential breath of life itself (as cited in Tolliver, 1997).

While spirituality is inherently and universally present within all human experience (O'Rourke, 1997; Tolliver,1997, Vaughan, 1991), the sense of being separate from or ignorant of spirit causes suffering (See next section). Thus, spirituality is subjectively experienced and usually described in terms of pursuit. It has been understood as an awareness or consciousness that must be cultivated as an aspect of human development (Derezotes, 1995). Maslow felt that spirituality is a human need to be fulfilled as the most advanced aspect of human development (Sermabeikian, 1994). Jung found that within each individual the human psyche has the capacity to metamorphize from instinctual to spiritually aware states of being (Sermabeikian, 1994). Spirit and psyche have often been viewed as synonymous. The word "psyche", which is the root of psychology, is derived from the Greek word *psukhe,* which means breath, life, soul. In ancient Greece, psyche was associated with spiritual dimensions of human nature and with femininity, beauty, and life (Elkins,1995; Sermabeikian, 1994).

Spiritual awareness has been described in terms of "…divinely focused altered states of consciousness" (Bullis, 1996, p.3). Vaughan (1991) mentions "…awareness of a transcendental dimension" (p. 105). Some feel that spirituality is experienced through the psyche, or the soul, which is thought of as a port or conduit for spirit. Accessing spirit through the soul is to connect to energy, essence, and vitality, and according to Jung the collective unconscious (Tolliver, 1997; Sermabeikian, 1994; McNiff, 1992).

Canda (1997) describes a human potentiality for spiritual wholeness, associating spirituality with inherent dignity, integrity, and completeness of every human being. Bloomfield describes spiritual wellness, which is experienced as a sense of fulfillment, satisfaction, peace, and unification or intimacy with God or nature (as cited by Tolliver, 1997). Tolliver (1997) goes on to describe this unification as the experience of "renewable life force, the energy that enlivens the physical and the space where human communion takes place' (p. 179). Tolliver (1997) further describes a potentiality for a spiritually imbued consciousness, which is experienced as profound connectedness. To experience spirituality is to commune with one's own nature, one's community, one's natural environment, and the divine (Canda, 1997; O'Rourke, 1997; Bullis, 1996; Griffith & Griffith, 1995; Moore, 1992). Within this connectedness, life is experienced as meaningful, sacred, and full (Vaughan, 1991).

Vaughan (1991) observed that spirituality can be experienced in diverse conditions and circumstance. For example, spirituality can be experienced in temples and churches, in nature, in art, in interpersonal relationships when one encounters death, and in every moment of our ordinary existence. Even those who reject the concept of the divine may experience life in a spiritual sense of connectedness with other human beings and with nature. This perspective has been called "humanistic spirituality" and also "phenomenological spirituality" (Lukoff, Lu & Turner, 1998). Furthermore, spirituality is expressed in many aspects of culture, including religion, art, and philosophy (Sermabeikian, 1994; McNiff, 1992).

It is not accurate to equate spirituality with religion. Religion is actually a compilation of beliefs and values through which individuals might relate to spirituality. These beliefs are codified and accepted by members of the religious community (Carroll, 1998; O'Rourke, 1997). Ideally, religion provides a reliable structure for spiritual practice. Yet, by institutionalizing spiritual experience, religions may tend to objectify and dogmatize spirituality. As Sermabeikian (1994) points out, confused beliefs can be institutionalized, which becomes very detrimental to individuals and to the community. He provides the examples of cults and hate groups. On the other hand, authentic spiritual connectedness is characterized by an aptitude for compassion and morality, which needs to be expressed within community (O'Rourke, 1997; Bullis, 1996; Vaughan, 1991).

Understanding Biopsychosocial Problems form a Spiritual Perspective

As the numbers of materially impoverished peoples increase globally, an increasingly small elite control much of the world's commerce, including media, food, energy, transportation, banking, and so on. For example, Monsanto, DuPont, and Novartis, who have a history of producing such products as toxic dyes, gunpowder, and saccharine, are competing to control 90% of the world's germ plasma. In doing so, they would control most of the world's food source. Economist Paul Hawkens calls this "the very opposite of the biological redundancy that is at the heart of ecosystem resilience and sustainability" (as cited by Pope , 2000, p. 43).

Furthermore, even among the wealthy, there is much unhappiness, frustration, quarreling, substance abuse, and even suicide (Watts, 1999; The Dalai Lama & Cutler, 1998). Modern culture holds to materialistic value, and thus, societies and individuals seek happiness through material gain. This ongoing pursuit of happiness through consumption never reaches a point of deep satisfaction; rather, consumers are always in the market for the next product or purchase. This is what fuels corporate greed. Watts (1999) describes how our modern culture of consumerism has resulted in hungry, insatiable societies that are exploiting our ecosystem to the point of destruction. He describes consumerism as the practice of unhappy people who are at a loss to compensate for a lack of meaning and pervasive anxiety regarding the human condition (Watts, 1999).

Pervasive anxiety and a sense of meaninglessness or inner void are underpinnings of world- wide biopsychosocial problems. This existential crises has been widely attributed to a lack of spiritual connectedness or spiritual poverty, sometimes called a loss of soul (Kellen -Taylor, 1998; Jaoudi, 1998; Russell, 1997; Elkins, 1995; Cowley & Derezotes, 1994; DuBray, 1993; Kurtz & Ketcham, 1992; McNiff, 1992; Moore, 1992). This spiritual poverty is evidenced by the great amount of spiritual seeking going on in our culture (Wuthnow, 1998; Elkins, 1995; Moore, 1992). Statistics show that a substantial number of Americans have lost confidence in our religious leaders (Lukoff, Lu & Turner, 1998). Many individuals are looking to other cultures for spiritual traditions and practices for guidance.

Russel (1997) describes spirituality as the unrealized potential of humanity. He finds that the pervasive suffering being experienced throughout modern society is due to the disconnection from the wisdom of this inner potential, which must be accessed as a foundation for sustainable and nondestructive behavior. Russell (1997) identifies a need to examine the underlying causes of today's global problems, and a need for a modern sacred path to facilitate their resolution. Cowley and Derezotes (1994) describe this "spiritual malaise" as evidenced by "value deficits, moral apathy, existential despair, spiritual emergencies and the like (p. 32). Violence has also been attributed to this spiritual lack (Watts, 1999; Ornish, 1997).

Modern culture worships independence and craves intimacy (The Dalai Lama & Cutler, 1998). Cardiologist and researcher Dr. Dean Ornish (1997) has identified what he calls "...emotional and spiritual heart disease–that is profound feelings of loneliness, isolation, alienation, and depression that are so prevalent in our culture..." (p. 12). Cutler also finds that there is a pervasive loneliness experienced in modern society (The Dalai Lama & Cutler, 1998). Substance abuse is a wide spread defense, another way to try to run away from this lack or feeling of inner "void" (Loy, 1992). Estelle (1990) describes the alienation which adolescents frequently suffer from, disabling their ability to individuate and mature. Feeling powerlessness can cause adolescents to distrust themselves, their families, and their communities. Ornish (1997) warns that historically, individuals and societies that practice nurturing and supportive behavior have had the greatest rates of survival, however, in our culture, time and energy spent nurturing each other is rapidly declining. Competition rather than nurturing is status quo.

Epstein (1995) refers to the problem as the narcissistic dilemma: "…the sense of falseness or emptiness that propels people either to idealize or to devalue themselves and others" (p. 6). There is an ongoing process which people get caught up in, that is the ongoing fabricating of our self image–the attempt to construct a desirable self and the self one thinks one should be, or at least appear to be. The dreams and disappointments of this striving is the hunger that drives over-consumption, exploitation, and violence in the name of self -interest (Watts, 1999; Chodron, 1997; Epstein, 1995 Loy, 1992).

People strive with great effort to be in control, but ultimately, this is impossible to achieve. Humans are acting like God want-to-be's, thinking that they can dictate reality. Ironically, this creates immense suffering, as individuals cannot live up to the expectation of making life what they want it to be.

There really is no place to hide from the ways of nature; the ultimate truths of life are greater than the concepts and desires of individuals. There is no lasting safe and profitable situation. Humanity's ongoing efforts to fabricate desirable selves in a desirable world are actually defenses to avoid what is the ultimate nature of all things, and a misinterpretation of the craving for spiritual wholeness (Chodron, 1997; Kurtz & Ketcham, 1992; Loy, 1992).

Finding Spirituality within Woundedness

Elkins (1995) explains that many psychologists recognize that psychopathology is frequently caused by spiritual lack, spiritual confusion, or spiritual conflict. Psychologists with this perspective include Erich Fromm, Irvin Yalom, Viktor Frankl, and Abraham Maslow. Elkins (1995) writes: "Psychopathology is the cry of our souls…the soul suffers when not nurtured by love… [it] will sustain woundedness if a person is deeply betrayed or abused. This creates psychopathology" (p. 91).

Grant (no date of publication cited) works extensively with survivors of trauma. He finds that traumatic experience can awaken spiritual awareness. He also describes the spiritual journey as a longing to align oneself to the power or vitality that sustains life, and emphasizes that often, individuals are forced through pain to let go of beliefs that are blinding them to their own spiritual consciousness. Grant refers to the stories of Jesus and of Buddha as examples of transformation through woundedness. He writes: "only by listening to our wounds can we live fully in spirit" (p. 5). Brennan (1993) attributes the woundedness that all humans have at their core to their perceived separateness from the boundless love of spiritual wholeness. The wound is like a well from which one can access creative energy, wisdom, and the beauty of essence, which is buried under many emotional and rationalized defenses. Remen (1996), describing the healing process of one of her clients who had been ashamed of her painful past writes: "Looking … at her woundedness, she found her power… [her] will to live…[her] courage, her ability to heal herself over and over again. Perhaps every victim is really a survivor who just doesn't know it yet" (p. 28). Albert Kreinheder summed it up when he wrote: "The greatest treasure comes out of the most despised and secret places… this place of greatest vulnerability is also a holy place, a place of healing…" (as cited in Duff, 1993).

Grant (no date) observed that the life process is marked by upheavals and continually challenging individuals to break out of self-judgment and rigid beliefs in order to deepen in spiritual awareness. He finds that the overall task of life itself is to transcend limited definitions of self, while aligning to that which is greater than self.

Even classic Western theorists recognize the role of upheaval and transformation in the process of maturation, a process which is inherent in the human experience. Freud's stages of psychosexual development are marked by trials and conflicts, which the child must master. In Erikson's model, each stage of psychosocial development is marked by a crises or conflict (Ashford, LeCroy & Lortie, 1997).

Thus, the process of psychosocial growth inevitably involves change via upheaval. Spiritual initiations have served in many cultures as rites of passage to facilitate and support individuals facing the painful transformations anticipated as part of the life process (Mason, 1996). However, in our culture, the custom is to avoid or deny one's vulnerabilities. Walsh (1996) associated modern biopsychosocial problems with psychological immaturity, due to the unwillingness in our culture to face uncomfortable truths. Death, for example, is one of the uncomfortable truths that is avoided, and not even discussed openly, in Western culture. Yet, the hardship of drawing close to death has the potentiality to open new doors to spiritual awareness (Chodron; 1997, Ardelt & Eichenberger-Levy, 1996; Remen, 1996; Vaughan, 1991).

Pain as a Tool for the Helping Professional

The pain social workers experience is comprised of feeling-level responses, or gut responses, to the biopsychosocial problems that we address. For social workers and other helping professionals, the synergy of self-aware, empathetic joining with the pain of clients, is the process by which we attain practice wisdom (Krill, 1990). By opening ourselves to the pain of others, we gain an intuitive understanding of the wounding that they are experiencing. In this way, we also cultivate empathy, sensitivity, and intuitive perceptiveness, which are *inner resources* that become tools for helping others (Rothman, 1999; Abramson, 1997; Sheafor, Horejsi & Horejsi, 1997; Krill, 1990). In order to do this, however, we must be willing to face our own pain as we "enter into the pain" of others (Sheafor, Horejsi & Horejsi, 1997, p. 37). Facing our own pain enhances our self-awareness and is often the vehicle for realizing our life's purpose (Grant, 1998; Brennan, 1993).

Helping professionals, such as social workers, often believe that they must distance themselves from their clients in order to take care of themselves, avoid enmeshment, and maintain the stature of an expert. However, while enmeshment takes place when there is confusion between the helper's needs and the client's needs, it is a misunderstanding to assume that being authentically present and profoundly receptive to the experience of the client on a gut level would imply such confusion. When a self-aware professional, who is willing to be personally impacted, changed, deeply touched, and moved by the ongoing predicaments of clients, be joining with the client or client system through this movement, and this can open both parties to new levels of trust, new perspectives, deeper understandings, and greater inner strengths. This authentic joining takes place within the discomfort of upheaval.

Spiritually rooted awareness is the key to effective social work practice and is a product of both our personal transformations and the joining of our transformational process with the transformational processes of our clients. This is something that each practitioner will accomplish in his or her own way and to different degrees. Extraordinary social work is born of this effort, and the greatest examples of this include the work of Mahatma Gandhi, Martin Luther King Jr., Nelson Mandela, Mother Teresa, and The Dalai Lama. Each of these individuals worked deeply with their personal spirituality, which facilitated their ability to impact society.

When helping professionals try to protect themselves by distancing their humanness, vulnerabilities, and "not knowing" from clients, their work loses its integrity. To illustrate how distancing one's inner can become a pitfall, I will relate an experience I had with a particular psychologist. Although she was not a social worker, she was a helping professional, who fell into the kind of trap that could happen to any of us.

In 1989, I was employed as a secretary by this psychologist who billed herself as an expert in cancer counseling. She had survived cancer, and her practice was based upon her own experience of recovery. During her illness, a particular doctor successfully treated her with an "alternative" medical regime. She also participated in a type of emotive group therapy, which was administered by a very charismatic psychotherapist, who had developed the method himself. I heard her frequently lecturing her clients, confidently describing how she had been cured by the synergy of these two treatments. She eloquently cited the latest scientific research in psychoneuroimmunology to validate the curative power of psychotherapy.

During the time I worked for her, this psychologist was diagnosed with a reoccurrence of cancer. Despite this, she continued to tell her therapy groups the same story of how she beat cancer, and she administered her prescription for cure while billing herself as an expert until she died. Part of my job was to assist in the therapy groups. During these groups, we paired up and did emotive work, venting our emotions with the support of our partners. I observed that she, herself, never participated and never expressed her emotions. In our private conversations, she also continued to espouse her expertise. I clumsily tried to find ways to address her current illness with her, but anything I said on the subject seemed to hurt her feelings.

This psychologist's expertise seemed to be like a castle built out of sand and dreams. She was certainly knowledgeable and an eloquent lecturer. However, her identity as an expert did not seemingly help her to face her vulnerability, her deep "not knowing", as she was compelled by her illness to transition to life's greatest mystery–death. Life and death are processes that cannot be controlled, not even by experts.

Some years later I ran into a young women, a cancer patient who had been a client of this psychologist. She expressed to me how angry, hurt, and confused she had felt because the psychologist had manipulated her. It seems that the client was providing emotional energy to support the psychologist during their sessions. I was not surprised to hear this. My impression was that in an effort to hold on to her expertise, the psychologist had isolated herself. Doing so hurt her and her client.

In Western culture, we often think that intellectual expertise and technology can place us above problems and upheaval, thereby making life secure. However, to ignore the transient nature of our lives is to ignore the mystery of our transpersonal spiritual essence. To ignore our vulnerability is delusional. Such denial causes *disconnectedness* from our own essence and the essence of our ecology, leading to the suffering of personal and existential isolation which is a state of spiritual poverty.

Use of Self in Spiritually Rooted Social Work

Chodron (1997) recommends that in the face of trials and upheaval one: "relax and touch the limitless space of the human heart" (Chodron, 1997, p. 59). Through this open, unguarded, completely relaxed embrace of being boundless joy is experienced. Obstacles can thus become opportunities to cultivate this unconditional acceptance. Enemies become teachers. By allowing one's life to be shaken, one touches the mind of "not knowing", not solving, not fixing, and not manipulating. This is touching the wisdom mind. This is to live fully while dying over and over again. Looking into one's own heart, one "discovers the universe" (Chodron, 1997, p. 75). One discovers that everybody and everything is awake, precious, and whole, and everyone experiences kinship with all beings. Then one can help others look into their hearts. In an open state of being, accepting whatever arises in every moment, one exudes a sense of peace and acceptance. Only in this openness, when letting go of all of the ego's agendas, can one fully experience who others really are. It is imperative to let our hearts be touched by suffering, which feels like touching an emotional wound. This openness is beyond bias, meaning one cannot make anything completely right or completely wrong. In this way, one cultivates compassion for self and for others. One must explore all aspects of oneself completely and nonjudgementally. One must fully experience one's own darkness and poisons. Then , knowing their painful nature, one can connect with every aspect of others, experiencing them fully and nonjudgementally, experiencing true compassion for them and for their confusion and pain with which they react to the groundlessness of being. Furthermore, "The real transformation takes place when we let go of our attachments and give away what we think we can't" (Chodron, 1997, p. 102). Relaxing and opening to whatever arises, one can give beyond one's perceived limits. In this process, one touches the groundless nature of all, and in doing so, one realizes that one is not stuck. The one can share this relief with others who are struggling. Chodron (1997)names Nelson Mandela, Mother Teresa, and the Dalai Lama as three mentors and examples of this process.

Conti-O'Hare (1998) finds that the experiencing of one's own woundedness enables one to find the healer within, for in this way one learns what heals and how to take part in the healing process. She describes how nurses discover that their own buried wounds can surface through their empathic feelings for the client's pain. This impacts their relationship with the client. The motivation to ease the pain of others is often birthed through one's own experience of pain which is real and raw. Conti-O'Hare (1998) uses the concept of the archetypical *Wounded Healer,* which originated in the mythic Greek figure called Chiron, who was a centaur (part horse, part man). Chiron had a painful, partially crippling, incurable wound. Through self-sacrifice, Chiron bore the pain of others and was able to heal them. Eventually, Chiron transcended his own pain by sacrificing his life in an act of compassion, which involved going to hell to save Prometheus from having to do so (Conti-O'Hare, 1998). Thus, the *Wounded Healer* cultivates the ability to exchange self-concern for selfless-compassion, and thus, transcends the duality of pain and pleasure–just as Jesus did when he died on the cross. his is also portrayed in the stories of the Buddhas and Bodhisattva (Chodron, 1997).

Grant (no date of publication cited), a therapist who works with traumatized clients, finds that by courageously surrendering one's own ego to
one's woundedness, wholeness, spiritual endowments, and healing abilities result. He describes that it is each individual's choice, whether to grasp
for security or deepen spiritually. Conti-O'Hare (1998) describes how
helping professionals, who can accesses their own woundedness as a conduit for empathetic joining with the pain of clients, are actually *Wounded
Healers*. *Wounded Healers* join with clients through their pain in this way,
causing a kind of sacred sharing or communion to take place which
enhanced the client's sense of wholeness and connectedness.

A lack of social relationship and spiritual connectedness creates profound isolation. Jourard writes: "every maladjusted person…has not
made himself known to another human being and in consequence does
not know himself…other people come to be stressors … in proportion to
his degree of self alienation" (as cited in Estelle, 1990, p.111). Art therapist, Shaun McKniff (1992), finds that he, himself, has experienced healing through the process of joining with the very clients he helps. He
writes: "the patients have also helped us, they have helped the soul, by
drawing our attention to its needs" (McKniff, 1992, p. 24). McKniff
(1992) points out that all humans are wounded, and he finds that pathology must be embraced as part of the experience of the soul. Mental health
practitioners are in denial if they think that the patient is sick and they are
not. When the staff realize their pathology, the system is ready for transformation. The concept of therapy is transformed by viewing the effort of
the patient and the therapist as expressions of the soul's purpose to heal
itself. This is our common purpose as humans, to "activate the resources of
the soul" (McKniff, 1992, p. 26).

Stiver (1990) also points out how mental health clients are starved for
intimacy, yet, their behavior patterns keep them from being able to have
satisfying relationships, a symptom of disconnectedness which causes
much suffering. In fact, research has shown that intimacy experienced in
support groups has prolonged the lives of breast cancer patients and even

reversed disease in the case of heart patients (Stein, 1999; Ornish, 1997). The love and caring shared in breast cancer support groups, the compassion and kindness of the doctor who was their facilitator, and the relief of not having to face the danger alone were reported as factors of primary importance by group members (Stein, 1999). Dr. Remen (1996) writes: "When we are seen by the heart we are seen for who we are... valued for our uniqueness ... we become able to know and value ourselves" (p. 149).

The process of deep joining is a compassionate and selfless act. Stiver (1990) is a psychotherapist who uses a relational model of therapy which acknowledges that both client and therapist will change as they touch each other through the therapeutic relationship. She describes her experiences of joining with clients through pain. She writes: "sometimes in therapy hour I found myself holding my breath, overwhelmed and overpowered by the pain... I knew each time I had moved a little further in my sense of community with others" (Stiver, 1990, p. 10). Elkins (1995) writes: "I can only be a healer of the soul when I am in contact with and reaching out with my own soul... the path to the client's soul begins in my own soul" (p. 92).

The path of the *Wounded Healer* embraces woundedness, and thus, eventually transcendence of the duality of joy and suffering through opening to woundedness coupled with compassionate work. In this way, healing becomes an instrument of transcendence or spiritual wholeness as one embraces groundlessness of their own wounds and opens their heart to selfless compassion for others (Cohen, 2000; Conti-O'Hare, 1998; Remen, 1996). Dr. Lawlis (1996) writes: "A strong, powerful sense of caring, a special kind of love from another being can provide the grace and energy for transformation... (and) our awareness of the infinite possibilities within each of us... reassures us that the mysteries of the universe are also altruistic" (p. 77).

Conti-O'Hare (1998) describes some of the dynamics of the path of the *Wounded Healer*. Initially, the desire to heal can grow from an effort to greater understand their own suffering, and, as the healers come to know

the healing value of their actions and insights, they can use these to benefit patients. However, this is possible only when the healers are able to
maintain a constant self- awareness and insight regarding their own pain
and their empathetic reactions in the moment, thus being able to avoid
any enmeshment or transference regarding the wounded client.
Additionally, the healers must apply clarity and insight to their understanding of the client's response to their healing relationship. Thus, the
client's inner healing is impacted by the helpers clarity, openness, and self-
awareness (Conti-O'Hare, 1998).

In terms of cultivation self-awareness, Cutler suggests: "take some time
to reflect on our own value system and reduce it to its fundamental principles… allows (will) us the greatest freedom and flexibility to deal with
the vast array of problems that confront us on a daily basis" (The Dalai
Lama & Cutler, 1998, p. 195). Bullis (1996) finds that the degree of self-
awareness needed in order to facilitate transformation and healing must be
maximized, therefore, it must be cultivated on an ongoing basis through
unflinching, honest self-examination, which is actually an initiation into
the transformational process through our own woundedness. Undergoing
this a process of this depth prepares the practitioner to cultivate the
potency to heal, and thus fulfilling the role of a modern day shaman or
psychopomp (Bullis, 1996).

As for cultivating openness, The Dalai Lama said: "If you maintain a
feeling of compassion, loving kindness, then something automatically
opens your inner door (The Dalai Lama & Cutler, 1998, p. 40). Clarity
occurs through openness in the moment and through the accessing of
intuitive, subconscious wisdom as well as intellectual knowledge (Lewis,
1997). Stiver (1990) finds that in order for the therapist to be truly
authentic and accessible in relationship with clients, the therapist must be
empathically and mutually involved in the therapeutic relationship by
being: ready to expose her vulnerabilities by being responsive and attuned,
cognitively and affectively, to what she experiences with the client. This

means the therapist is open to change" (p. 8). The client is thus empowered by this experience of truly touching and impacting another person.

Jung stated that one rarely finds an analyst who has the capacity to actually heal others, which can only be achieved through the analyst's own woundedness. He noted that vulnerability and wholeness are essential to this facilitate the healing process, rather than "clean hands perfection" (Conti-O'Hare, 1998). In modern culture, doctors have been taught to practice with "clean hands perfection", which has been dehumanizing and demoralizing for themselves and patients alike (Novack, Epstein, & Paulsen, 1999; Ornish,1997; Remen, 1996). There is a need to bring the magic and sacredness back to the healing relationship (Lawlis, 1996). It has been documented that so called remedies have been successfully used to treat illness even though they were useless or even harmful. In such cases, the doctor-patient relationship was the healing factor. Novack, et al. (1999) explain that healing involves communication. He remarks on the importance of offering clients: words of reassurance, affirmations, forgiveness; active listening , understanding of the patients' illness in the context of their life situation; trustworthiness; empathy and understanding, a sense of humor; and, occasional self-disclosures. Healing draws upon the healers' integrity, respect, and compassion. Emotional distancing in medical practice leads to: "burnout, addiction, and emotional impairment" (Novack, et al., 1999, 517).

Lewis (1997) reminds us of Jung once again, stating: "Jung had felt that unless both the analyzed and the analyst are healed no healing occurs" (p.24). Remen (1996), in her book *Kitchen Table Wisdom, Stories that Heal*, recounts many encounters with clients wherein she joined them in their pain in such a way that was healing and beneficial. Remen (1996) also tells her own story, which reveals how her own wounds have softened her, teaching her to open her heart to others. Through her extremely difficult struggle to come to terms with her own pain, Darlene Cohen (2000) has followed this path as well. She has suffered for twenty years with intense chronic pain. Through training her mind, she has actually found joy and has recently published her recent book: Finding a Joyful Life in the Heart of Pain. Cohen (2000) shares how pain and pleasure are interdependent, and how her experience of pain awakened her to joy she had not previously been aware of. Cohen (2000), who once could not walk, now counsels chronic pain clients and lectures and teaches about pain management. She and Dr. Rachel Naomi Remen have both come to realize the same paradoxical actuality. As Remen (1996) states that the part in us that feels suffering is the same as the part that feels joy.

Perhaps the greatest acts of compassion are achieved through woundedness. The world's greatest spiritual figures, such as Jesus, embody compassion by offering their own welfare for the sake of others. Thus Jesus, wounded and dying on the cross, promised: "Fear not, I am with you" (Jaoudi, 1998, p. 109). Brennan's (1993) points out that all humans have wounds. She finds that the wounds are caused by the perception that self is separate from God. Through penetrating the wounds, one becomes connected to one's central core, creative process, gifts, and God's all pervasive love. Removing all blockages is humanity's life task. In doing so, one manifests one's life's work. What ever this life's work is, it will be healing for individuals, society, or both, for it will be divinely inspired and attuned. In this way, all people are potentially wounded healers (Brennan, 1993). Dr. Martin Luther King, Jr. said: "What does not destroy me, makes me stronger" (The Dalai Lama & Cutler, 1998, p. 201).

Just as the shamans are stung by a shattering experience which initiate them into their role, and as the *Hero* receives a "call" by an unsettling event, the archetypal *Wounded Healer* is wounded. The *Wounded Healers'* life's work chooses them. Conti-O'Hare (1998) find, for example, that a: "doctor knows, even unconsciously, that he did not chose this profession by chance and must come to terms with why he chose the profession (p. 17). Coming to terms with one's journey is central to the experience of living. Miller (1994) quotes Gabrial Marcel, who said: "the deeper we go within ourselves, the more we find of that which is beyond ourselves" (p. 58). Chodron (1997) writes: "Only to the extent that we expose ourselves over and over to annihilation can that which is indestructible be found in us" (p.7). Remen (1996) and Chodron (1997) add that it is essential to practice gentleness when going through this process. Opening one's heart means being kind to oneself, as well as others. For example, grieving is a part of this caring, and it must be acknowledged within oneself by a *Wounded Healer*. Dr. Remen also refers to self-care as "the antidote to professionalism" (p. 53). In addition, health care providers could enter into resonant, healing relationships with each other (Lawlis, 1996).

Extraordinary Social Work

Jaoudi (1998) finds that individuals have a mystical social gift to give, revealed to them in their prayer life. Bogart (1994) refers to this as "vocation". He describes vocation as one's pivotal life task and finds that discovering one's vocation is literally an initiation to realizing one's life purpose. Vocation is the spiritual journey–the *Hero's* risky quest. Bogart (1994) finds that three human necessities drive vocation: 1) the need for participating socially in a meaningful way; 2) the need to realize one's potentiality; and, 3) the essential connecting with spiritually aware guidance, even perhaps divine guidance. Bogart (1994) describes vocation as: "a unifying story that brings together the social, individual, and the sacred... that can be used to guide psychospiritual growth..."(p. 11-12). Vocation becomes a bridge between inner and outer worlds.

Vocation is a formula for extraordinary social work. In order for social work to become a path to spiritual healing, and in order to approach the work as a *Wounded Healer*, it would have to be more than a job. It would have to be a calling. There are plenty of biopsychosocial problems calling out to be addressed, tapping humanity on the shoulder and sometimes knocking humanity over the head. Park (1996) urges social workers to heed the call of global biopsychosocial problems, pointing out that pollution alone could destroy the entire ecosystem if there are not positive changes in the next ten years. She writes: "The social worker professional's call is to witness this crisis in a unique and creative way that will integrate the Earth into the center of our psychosocial lives" (Park, 1996, p. 320).

Extraordinary social work, then, is a *Hero's* journey, for it is a profession of individuals who set out to make a difference, to heal wounds, and to spend every day of their career addressing problems, crises, and upheaval without bombs and guns, without medical equipment, even without a Ph.D. and a fancy office. The social worker's primary tool is self (Sheafor, Horejsi & Horejsi, 1997). Buechner's description of the social worker's vocation seems especially poignant. He describes the vocation of social work as a "place where your deep gladness and the world's deep hunger meet"; this place is described as one of the "hospitality" of the social worker, "a space for others to continue their journey toward wholeness (as cited in Jacobs, 1997, p. 174).

References

Ardelt, M. & Eichenberger-Levy, S. 1996. *In Search for Meaning: The Role of Religion for Cancer Patients*. Paper presented to the American Sociological Association from the Department of Sociology, University of Florida, Gainesville, Florida, (352) 392- 0251, *ardelt@soc.ulf.edu.*

Ashford, J. B., LeCroy, C. W., & Lortie, K. L. 1997. *Human Behavior in the Social Environment: A Multidimensional Perspective.* Pacific Grove, California: Brooks/Cole Publishing Company.

Bogort, G. 1994. "Finding A Life's Calling". *Journal of Humanistic Psychology, 34* (4), 37.

Brennan, B. A. 1993. *Light Emerging: The Journey of Personal Healing.* New York: Bantom Books.

Bullis, R. K. 1996. *Spirituality in Social Work Practice.* Washington, DC: Taylor & Francis.

Canda, E. R. 1997. Spirituality. In R. L. Edwards (Eds.). *The Encyclopedia of Social Work* (19th Edition). Washington, DC: The National Association of Social Workers Press.

Canda, E. R. 1997. Does Religion and Spirituality Have A Significant Place in the Core HBSE Curriculum? Yes. In M. Bloom and W. C. Klein (Eds). *Controversial Issues in Human Behavior in the Social Environment.* Needham Heights, Massachusetts: Allyn & Bacon.

Carroll, M. M. 1998. Social Work's Conceptualization of Spirituality. In E. R. Canda (Ed.). *Spirituality in Social Work: New Directions.* (1-13). Binghamton, New York: The Hawthorn Pastoral Press.

Chodron, P. 1997. *When Things Fall Apart*. Boston: Shambhala Publications, Inc.

Cohen, D. 2000. *Find A Joyful Life in the Heart of Pain*. Boston: Shambhala Publications, Inc.

Conti-O'Hare, M. 1998. "Examining the Wounded Healer Archetype: A Case Study in Expert Addictions Nursing Practice". *Journal of American Psychiatric Nurses Association, 4* (3), 71-76.

Cowley, A., & Derezotes, D. 1994. "Transpersonal Psychology and Social Work Education". *Journal of Social Work Education, 30* (1), 32 - 41.

Dalai Lama, H. H., & Cutler, H. C. 1998. *The Art of Happiness*. New York: Riverhead Books.

DuBray, W. 1993. *Mental Health Interventions with People of Color*. St. Paul, Minnesota: West Publishing Company.

Duff, K. 1993. *The Alchemy of Illness*. New York: Bell Tower/ Crown Publishers, Inc.

Elkins, D. N. 1995. "Psychotherapy and Spirituality: Toward a Theory of the Soul". *Journal of Humanistic Psychology, 35* (2), 78-98.

Epstein, M. 1995. *Thoughts without A Thinker: Psychotherapy from A Buddhist Perspective*. New York, NY: Basic Books.

Estelle, C. J. 1990. "Contrasting Creativity and Alienation in Adolescent Experience". *The Arts and Psychotherapy, 17*, 109-115.

Grant, R. No date cited. *The Way of the Wound. Published by Robert Grant*: Burlingame, California: R. Grant.

Griffith, M. E., & Griffith, J. L. *1995. Opening Therapy to Sacred Conversations*. Paper Presented at the Third Annual International

Conference of Narrative Ideas & Therapeutic Practice. (March).Vancouver, British Columbia: Canada.

Jacobs, C. 1997. "Essay on Spirituality and Social Work Practice". *Smith College Studies in Social Work, 67 (2),* 171-175.

Jaoudi, M. 1998. *Christian Mysticism East and West: What the Masters Teach Us.* Mahwah, New Jersey: Paulist Press.

Kellen-Taylor, M. 1998. "Imagination and the World: A Call for Ecological Expressive Therapies". *The Arts in Psychotherapy,* 25(5), 303-311.

Krill, D. F. 1990. *Practice Wisdom: A Guide for Helping Professionals.* Newbury Park, California: Sage Publications.

Kurtz, E., & Ketchum, K. 1992. *The Spirituality of Imperfection: Storytelling and the Journey to Wholeness.* New York: Bantam Books.

Lawliss, G. F. 1996. *Transpersonal Medicine: A New Approach to Healing Body, Mind and Spirit.* Boston: Shambhala Publications, Inc.

Lewis, P. 1997. "Transpersonal Arts Psychotherapy: Toward an Ecumenical World View". *The Arts and Psychotherapy,* 24(3), 243-245.

Loy, D. 1992. "Avoiding the Void: The Lack of Self in Psychotherapy and Buddhism". *The Journal of Transpersonal Psychology,* 24(2), 151-179.

Lukoff, D., Lu, F., & Turner, R. 1998. "From Spiritual Emergency to Spiritual Problem: The Transpersonal Roots of the New DSM-IV Category". *Journal of Humanistic Psychology,* 38(2), 21-50.

Mason, M. J. 1996. "Family Therapy as Initiation: More than A Therapeutic Metaphor". *Journal of Family Psychotherapy,* 7(3) 31-38.

McKniff, S. 1992. *Art as Medicine: Creating A Therapy of the Imagination.* Boston: Shambhala Publications, Inc.

Miller, J. P. 1994. "Contemplative Practice in Higher Education: An Experiment in Teacher Development". *Journal of Humanistic Psychology, 34*(4), 53-69.

Moore, T. 1992. *Care of the Soul.* New York: Harper Collins Publishers, Inc.

Novack, D. H., Epstein, R. M., & Paulson, R. H. 1999. "Toward Creating Physician- healers: Fostering Medical Students' Self-awareness, Personal Growth, and Well-being". *Academic Medicine, 74*(5), 516-520.

Ornish, D. 1997. *Love and Survival: The Scientific Basis for the Healing Power of Intimacy.* New York: Harper Collins Publishers, Inc.

O'Rourke, C. 1997. "Listening for the Sacred: Addressing Spiritual Issues in the Group Treatment of Adults with Mental Illness". *Smith College Studies in Social Work, 67*(2), 177-196.

Park, K. M. 1996. "The Person is Ecological: Environmentalism of Social Work". Social Work, 41(3), 320-323.

Pope, C. 2000. "Getting it Right". (January/February). *Sierra,* 40-47.

Remen, R. N. 1994. *Kitchen Table Wisdom: Stories that Heal.* New York: Riverhead Books.

Rothman, J. C. 1999. *The Self-awareness Workbook for Social Workers.* Boston: Allyn & Bacon.

Russel, P. 1997. An Inner Manhattan Project. In B. Cortright (Ed.). *Psychotherapy and Spirit: Theory and Practice in Transpersonal Psychotherapy.* (252-253). Albany, New York: State University of New York Press.

Sermabeikian, P. 1994. "Our Clients, Ourselves: The Spiritual Perspective and Social Work Practice". *Social Work, 39*(2), 178-183.

Sheafor, B. W., Horejsi, C.R., & Horejsi, G. 1997. *Techniques and Guidelines for Social Work Practice.* (Revised Edition). Boston: Allyn and Bacon.

Stein, L. 1999. "Prescription Hope: Stanford Psychologist David Spiegel Walks the Line between Mind and Body, Medicine and Psychology. (April 14). *Palo Alto Weekly,* 18-21.

Stiver, I. P. 1989. *Dysfunctional Families and Wounded Relationships: Part I.* Paper Presented at a Stone Center Colloquium. (May 3). Boston: Wellesley College.

Stiver, I. P. 1989. *Dysfunctional Families and Wounded Relationships: Part II.* Paper Presented at a Stone Center Colloquium. (November 1). Boston: Wellesley College.

Tolliver, W. 1997. "Invoking the Spirit: A Model for Incorporating the Spiritual Dimension of Human Functioning into Social Work Practice". *Smith College Studies in Social Work, 67*(3), 177-186.

Vaughan, F. 1991. "Spiritual Issues in Psychotherapy". *The Journal of Transpersonal Psychology, 23*(2), 105-119.

Walsh, R. 1996. Toward a Psychology of Human and Ecological Survival: Psychological Approaches to Contemporary Global Problems. In B. W. Scotten, A. B. Chinen, and J. R. Battista (Eds.). *Textbook of Transpersonal Psychiatry and Psychology.* (396-405). New York: Basic Books.

Watson, K. W. 1994. "Spiritual Emergency: Concepts and Implications for Psychotherapy". *Journal of Humanistic Psychology*, 34(2), 22-45.

Watts, J. 1999. *The First Noble Truth (Dukkha): The Spiritual Roots and Delusions of Consumer Culture*. (January 13). [WWW document]. URL *http://www.igc.apc.org/bpt/watts1.html*.

Wuthnow, R. 1998. "Morality, Spirituality, and Democracy". *Society*, 35(3) 37-45.

Chapter 8

Forgiveness and Healing

Wynne DuBray

Forgiveness is one of the main tenets of Christianity, as was recently demonstrated when Pope John Paul II took the extraordinary step of asking for forgiveness of the Roman Catholic Church for the sins and crimes committed in the name of Christ against the Jews, indigenous peoples, and many others. This was not only a critical moment in history, but also a major step toward healing.

In the Bible, Matthew 5:43-44 states: "You have heard that it hath been said, Thou shalt love thy neighbor, and hate thine enemy. ...But I say unto you, Love your enemies, bless them that curse you, do good to them that hate you, and pray for them which despitefully use you, and persecute you". Here the scripture states that intelligent love, which comprehends the difficulty and extends itself to rescue the enemy from his hate, is akin to God's loving action toward rebellious men and, thus, is a demonstration that those who so love are true sons of their Father. There are many examples of forgiveness in the Bible, but, perhaps the most dramatic and profound passage is the statement of Jesus on his cross of crucifixion, Luke 23:34, when He says: "Father, forgive them for they know not what they do".

Forgiveness As A Psychological Intervention

Forgiveness may be conceived of as either a spiritual/religious principle or as a "secular, individualized psychosocial construct"(Thoresen, 2000). Christianity does not have a monopoly on forgiveness; it is not religious property. Forgiveness applies to every human being, whether one is a Muslim, a Jew, or an atheist. Misunderstandings and hurt are a basic part of all relationships and forgiveness is necessary to restore these relationships. Forgiveness is to give up resentment and start over again with a clean slate. Types of forgiveness include: forgiving another with whom one no longer has a relationship; forgiving another with whom one has an ongoing relationship; seeking forgiveness from another for one's own transgressions; and, self-forgiveness.

The value of forgiveness, however, is much broader than to restore a relationship. Its effects can be profound and miraculous. When people are hurt or injured, they usually respond with anger and want to get revenge. Revenge keeps the wound open, and it cannot be healed. Staying stuck in negative feelings drains one's energy and usually leads to depression and sometimes even physical illness. Forgiveness can help a person become free from this anger and to move on with his/her life.

Unfortunately, forgiveness is not always possible, especially for victims of violent crimes. Some people can, however, work through those feelings and focus on other more positive goals in life, without forgiving those who have harmed them. For example, many victims of sexual assault have focused on helping other victims and have become empowered by their activities in helping others. Waiting for some justice or redress, that may never come, is often counterproductive.

Forgiveness costs something when one is angry and wants revenge. The desire for revenge can be deadly, leading to alcoholism, depression, and other physical disorders. Forgiveness requires one to surrender one's pride or one's desire for revenge. Some people feel that the other person will continue to feel guilty if they fail to forgive that person, thus they will have power over the other person to punish him or her. The other person may never ask for forgiveness or take responsibility for his or her actions. Therefore, the victim must decide whether to let go of his or her anger and stop allowing the incident to upset him or her.

Family members of murder victims report that they feel no satisfaction at the execution of the murderer. They are relieved that the murderer cannot harm any other people, but there is no release of their pain when another person is put to death.

Forgiveness and Psychotherapy

According to Malcolm and Greenberg (2000), there are five theoretical components of forgiveness. These components are as follows:

1. Acceptance into awareness of strong emotions such as anger and sadness;
2. Letting go of previously unmet interpersonal needs;
3. Shift in the forgiving person's view of the offender;
4. Development of empathy for the offender; and,
5. The construction of a new narrative of self and other.

Forgiveness is a key component in psychotherapy, especially in working with couples in relationship therapy. It is important for couples to forgive each other on a daily basis in order to live together in peace and harmony.

Forgiveness as an element in therapy, however, has not generated much impact on research and practice (McCullough & Worthington, 1994). Forgiveness is frequently addressed in pastoral counseling as a major component (Jeff, 1987; Leech, 1994; Lyall, 1995). Unfortunately, one of the key limitations of social work practice is the lack of recognition of the key role of forgiveness in psychological healing.

Enright (1996) examined forgiveness in three aspects: forgiving others; forgiving self; and, receiving forgiveness. The spiritual beliefs of the social worker/therapist involved determines, to a great extent, whether forgiveness will be addressed in the therapeutic process (DiBlasio & Proctor, 1993). One must be cautious in encouraging premature forgiveness in cases where the client has not been sufficiently supported in working through anger and other feelings involved. A Christian approach can move too quickly into forgiveness (McNeice, 1996). Richards and Bergin (1997)point out: "When people attempt to forgive prematurely, the healing process is prevented from occurring, and invalidated and unresolved feelings of pain, grief, guilt, shame, anger, and rage continue to create problems for them in their lives" (p. 213).

Encouraging forgiveness is one of the most frequently used spiritual interventions by psychotherapists (Richards & Bergin, 1997). Forgiveness, in order to be effective and healing, needs to be carried out by clients in their own time. The sense of hurt and damage is so great for some clients that forgiveness cannot be achieved.

When people have been emotionally hurt, it is important to remember that much abusive behavior and verbal abuse is a projection of the speaker's own hurts and psychological makeup. Much of human behavior stems from unconscious motivation and drives. Once this behavior is recognized as projection and displacement, it is much easier to forgive.

Forgiving oneself is a major problem for people who have grown up in a guilt based family system. These individuals have unrealistic expectations of themselves and measure themselves by a perfect standard. Many substance abusers suffer from guilt due to past behavior when they were under the influence of drugs or alcohol. Following the twelve-step program helps these clients to work through the guilt and, at times, make restitution for past misdeeds.

Kurtz and Ketcham (1994) state that to forgive involves letting go of the feeling of resentment (whether toward self or others) and of the vision that underlies that feeling—the vision in which we see ourselves as being offended against, or the vision of self-as-victim. The main spiritual shift that takes place in the event of being forgiven/forgiving is a new experiencing of self. Blaming others falls away, and we begin to accept primary responsibility for who we are. Forgiveness comes when we let go of the feeling of resentment by surrendering the vision of self-as-victim. If we have been injured, we no longer experience the injury as a barrier to relationship. Instead, we see the injury in the perspective of our own imperfection. How can we expect anyone else to be perfect if we ourselves are imperfect? Kurtz and Ketcham (1994) summarize this: "Thus it is that we do not forgive; instead, we discover forgiveness in both its forms–both that we have been forgiven and that we have forgiven. Spirituality's mutuality holds true here as everywhere: We are forgiven only if we are open to forgiving, but we are able to forgive only in being forgiven–we get only by giving, and we give only be getting" (p. 222).

Advantages of Forgiveness

Preliminary research on forgiveness shows that patients who move toward forgiving someone who has wronged them show decreases in anxiety and depression(Sanderson & Linehan, 1999). Research also shows that "defensive responses such as revenge fantasies and blaming have been associated with psychopathology…and poor health outcomes"(Exline & Baumeister, 2000, p. 134). Furthermore, research demonstrates that "forgiveness can be an important step in restoring relationships that have been harmed through transgression" (Exline & Baumeister, 2000, p. 150). All of this contributes greatly to the personal healing process of clients.

Potential Disadvantages of Forgiveness

There are a number of disadvantages to forgiveness that have been articulated by clients. These include the following:

1. Victims fear that forgiveness will give the perpetrator free license to repeat the transgression.
2. This may keep the victim in a destructive relationship.
3. Victims fear appearing weak or vulnerable.
4. The victims hold the belief that justice will not be served.

5. Loss of benefits of victim status, such as occupying the high moral ground or having the power to induce guilt, to demand reparations, or to punish the perpetrator (Exline & Baumeister, 2000: Pargament, McCullough & Thoresen, 2000).

Problems with Empirical Studies of Forgiveness

There are problems with empirical studies of forgiveness. According to Malcolm and Greenberg, these problems include the following:

1. Research is still in the preliminary stages.
2. Studies have shown that psychoeducational programs can promote forgiveness; however, most studies used self-selected samples rather than clinical samples.
3. Models of forgiveness have not been validated: general therapeutic factors may account for positive results, rather than the theorized components or steps to forgiveness.

Application of Social Work Practice

Spiritual approaches, such as interventions involving forgiveness, have been foreign for social workers, even though they have been pioneers in helping individuals become liberated from psychic pain for many years. The making of conscious choices that lead to proactivity instead of reactivity is one of the components of spiritual empowerment.

Many social workers were reluctant to address spirituality with clients, as it was considered the domain of the spiritual leaders in organized churches. Transpersonal psychology and the work of Carl Jung, along with twelve-step programs in the treatment of addiction, have been the major foci of services that could be considered spiritual approaches of social work practice.

The non-existence of universal models to help social workers deal with spiritual issues continues to be a challenge. Many social workers report that the pressure of brief therapy required by managed care requirements leads to "burn-out" and feelings of impotence in meeting the client's needs. Spiritual approaches can help clients become aware that they are responsible for creating their world and their experiences in life.

Case Examples

The author, having worked with over a thousand couples in relationship therapy, has seen hundreds of examples of healing of relationships once the couple can forgive each other for harmful and hurtful events in the relationship and begin each day with the intention of making the relationship work. In some instances, there has been infidelity and unfaithfulness on the part of one or both partners. When forgiveness is possible, the relationship is usually healed. On the other hand, there are some people who are not able to forgive, and punishment and/or revenge are usually the motives. In these cases, the relationship is usually over, and the partners go their separate ways. In this section, a number of case examples are provided to demonstrate the use of forgiveness.

Case of Mary and John

Mary had grown up as an only child and was accustomed to having a lot of attention. She was not used to sharing with others, and she was lacking in social skills. John was one of ten children, being the second to the youngest in the family. In this relationship, John was forgiving of hurtful behaviors in the relationship. However, Mary was not able to forgive and held grudges over minor short-comings of John's. Once Mary became aware of how much unnecessary pain she was inflicting upon herself, she was able to learn how to forgive, and she experienced the freedom that comes with this. Hence, the relationship was saved, and the couple continued to grow in their love and commitment to each other.

Case of Lynn

Lynn was the mother of a fifteen year old daughter, who was gang raped by four high school males that were minors. They were not punished for this vicious crime and were placed on a few months probation. Lynn was very bitter and wanted revenge, since she felt that justice was not served. For two years, she carried this rage and anger with her until the emotional and physical health of both herself and her family became jeopardized. Lynn finally sought counseling from a spiritually oriented social worker, who suggested that she try forgiving these males through prayer and leaving the judgement up to the Great Spirit. Lynn was able to let go of her anger and rage through prayer and experienced the miracle of freedom and healing through forgiveness. She was finally able to get on with her life and to become a functioning human being once again.

The Brown Family

The Brown Family was a family that thrived on conflict. At family gatherings, it was not unusual to have at least one or two family quarrels between family members, which resulted in several members not speaking to each other for long periods of time. A crisis occurred when, at the funeral of the grandfather, an argument between two sons developed into a fist fight with both being arrested for assault and battery. The wives of the two brothers contacted a social worker to conduct an intervention/healing exercise which would unite the family so the funeral services could proceed.

The social worker met with the family and led an exercise of self examination and forgiveness, which was welcomed by the family. This social worker had additional sessions with the family, which led to greater unity and less bickering at family gatherings.

Micro, Mezzo, and Macro Levels

The above cases are primarily at the level of micro social work. Much of the exercises in conflict resolution at the mezzo levels can incorporate forgiveness with great promise. Staff retreats can utilize spiritual models of forgiveness to bring employees together and create harmony in the work place. At the macro level, entire communities have utilized forgiveness and restoration/restitution in the aftermath of war crimes in Africa. The Sun Dance of the Lakota incorporates forgiveness in bringing together the entire community for unity and thanksgiving on an annual basis. Chapter 10 of this text addresses this in greater depth.

Summary and Conclusion

This chapter has addressed forgiveness and healing as they relate to social work practice at the micro, mezzo and macro levels. Forgiveness is not always possible, nor is it indicated in some cases, and social workers are cautioned to examine the appropriateness of these interventions with each case. Research on forgiveness, as it is applied in mental health settings, is very limited. In instances where the harm is extreme, and the trauma devastating, other approaches to healing, growth, and empowerment may be more effective.

References

DiBlasio, F. A., & Proctor, J. H. 1993. "Therapists and the Clinical Use of Forgiveness". *American Journal of Family Therapy, 21* (2), 175-83.

Enright, D. 1996. "Counseling Within the Forgiveness Triad: On Forgiving, Receiving Forgiveness, and Self-forgiving". *Counsel and Values, 40* (2), 107-26.

Exline, J. J., & Baumeister, R. F. 2000. "Expressing Forgiveness and Repentance: Benefits and Barriers. In M. E. McCullough, K. I. Pargament, and C. E. Thoresen (Eds.). *Forgiveness: Theory, Research, and Practice* (pp. 133-155). New York: Guilford.

Iversen Associates. 1972. *The New Testament and Wycliffe Bible Commentary.* (Third Edition). New York: Moody Monthly.

Jeff, M. 1987. *Spiritual Direction for Every Christian.* London: SPCK.

Kurtz, E., & Ketcham, K. 1994. *The Spirituality of Imperfection.* (Second Edition).New York: Bantam Books.

Leech, K. 1994. *Soul Friend.* London: Darton, Longman and Todd.

Lyall, D. 1995. *Counseling in the Pastoral and Spiritual Context.* Buckingham: Open University Press.

Malcolm, W. M., & Greenberg, L. S. 2000. Forgiveness as A Process of Change in Individual Psychotherapy. In M. E. McCullough, K. I. Pargament, and C. E. Thoresen (Eds.). *Forgiveness: Theory, Research, and Practice* (pp. 179-203). New York: Guilford.

McCullough, M. E., & Worthington, E. L. 1994. "Models of Interpersonal Forgiveness and Their Application to Counseling: Review and Critique". *Counseling and Values, 39* (1), 2-14.

McNeice, M. (1996) "Premature forgiveness", *Self & Society, 24* (2), 11-13.

Pargament, K. I., McCullough, M. E., & Thoresen, C. E. 2000. The Frontier of Forgiveness: Seven Directions for Psychological Study and Practice. In M. E. McCullough, K. I. Pargament, and C. E. Thoresen (Eds.). *Forgiveness: Theory, Research, and Practice* (pp.299-320). New York: Guilford.

Richards, P. S., & Bergin, A. E. 1997. *A Spiritual Strategy for Counseling and Psychotherapy*. Washington, DC: American Psychological Association.

Sanderson, C., & Linehan, M. M. 1999. Acceptance and Forgiveness. In W. R. Miller (Ed.). *Integrating Spirituality into Treatment: Resources for Practitioners* (pp. 199-216). Washington, DC: American Psychological Association.

Thoresen, C. E. 2000. Forgiveness and Health: An Unanswered Question. In M. E. McCullough, K. I. Pargament, and C. E. Thoresen (Eds.). *Forgiveness: Theory, Research, and Practice* (pp. 254-280). New York: Guilford.

Chapter 9

Spirituality and Mental Health

Wynne DuBray

Why is there such an interest in spirituality in our society today? The timing seems to be right for practitioners, such as social workers, to incorporate spiritual approaches into the delivery of mental health services. Could it be that baby boomers are aging, triggering questions about the meaning of life in the face of disability and death? Could it be that people feel disconnected today, even within their own families and communities? Could it be that we, as consumers, are sick and tired of the relentless search for material forms of happiness? Could it be that we live in an age of narcissism? Are we at last questioning our quest for super achievement, blind ambition, and workaholism? As "rugged individuals", do we feel a low-grade alienation, even from ourselves? Although Americans' earnings, adjusted for inflation, have more than doubled since 1957, our level of happiness has remained flat, and rates of depression have soared (Myers, 2000).

History teaches us that alienation of individualism leads to a thirst for spiritual and religious community. History also teaches us that there are limits of psychotherapy and medication as solutions to life's problems. One must also acknowledge that there are limits of science, reason, or politics as the answer to life's problems.

Multiculturalism, as an essential perspective in clinical social work, views religion and a spiritual world view as major parts of a client's cultural world

(Worthington, Kuruso, McCullough & Sandage, 1996). Spirituality is of utmost importance in the lives of people from all cultures and, in many cases, cannot be separated from their religious beliefs and/or philosophy of life.

Definitions of Spirituality and Religion

The terms spirituality and religion must be clearly understood, as they have different meanings. Religion is the search for meaning and purpose in ways related to the sacred. Here, *sacred* means higher powers, transcendent forces, or personal beings (Pargament, 1992). Most religions claim to be moral by promoting behavior that is right, just, and good.

Spirituality, on the other hand, cannot be easily defined, but most definitions include references to motivation and experience (Thoresen, 1999).

The motivation, to seek meaning and purpose in ways not necessarily related to the *sacred* and the transcendent, unitive, or transpersonal experience, gives us a sense of connecting beyond our individual selves. Spirituality may or may not involve the *sacred*. It can be a form of expressing one's creativity. Such experiences are amoral: a person's experience of self-transcendence may be what others would regard as good or evil. Spiritual experience can have an exposure to both positive and negative energy. Whether a spiritual experience is deemed good, bad, or neutral depends upon how one evaluates the meaning and values that frame it.

In defining spirituality, some people focus more on observable, moral behaviors, especially love: "spirituality I take to be concerned with those qualities of the human spirit–such as love and compassion, patience, tolerance, forgiveness, contentment, a sense of responsibility, a sense of harmony–which bring happiness to both self and others"(The Dalai Lama, 1999, p. 22). There is a great deal of overlap between spirituality and religion. Spirituality may include religion, but it is a broader concept. Spirituality includes a sense of oneness with others and numinous experiences (Otto, 1970). One can experience a sense of wonder when contemplating a *sacred being*, with the sense that the self is nothing by comparison. Almond (1982) states that spiritual experiences can be described as a "mysteriousness" that is both awful and dreadful; yet, it is also fascinating and compelling. Mystical experiences are usually accompanied by feelings of peace, awareness of the *sacred*, and a sense that the experience cannot be described in words. Usually there is a sense of oneness with a *sacred being*, or a cosmic consciousness, a sense of being one with all things, animate or inanimate (Newberg & D'Aquili, 1998).

Mystical Experiences

How common are mystical and numinous experiences? American Indians report numerous examples of mystical and numinous experiences(DuBray,1999). Researchers have surveyed the general population with questions, such as the following:

1. Would you say that you have ever had a "religious or mystical experience"–that is, a moment of sudden religious awakening or insight?
2. Have you ever felt as though you were close to a powerful spiritual force that seemed to lift you out of yourself?
3. Have you ever been aware of or influenced by a presence or power, whether you call it God or not, which is different from your everyday self?

Overall, about 35-40% of respondents report having these numinous or mystical experiences. Other findings include:

1. Women report more of these experiences than men.
2. The experiences tend to increase in frequency with age.
3. They are characteristic of the educated and affluent.
4. Subjects reporting these experiences are healthier psychologically.
5. Those who have these experiences rarely tell others about them.

Spirituality includes both numinous experiences, as well as "spirituality of everyday life", such as expressing love for humanity and for all living creatures (Hood, Spilka, Hunsberger, & Gorsuch, 1996, p. 245-7).

Assessment of Spirituality

In applying spiritual interventions in social work practice, one can use a variety of approaches. The assessment should include the following at minimum:

1. Identifying stress buffers: sources of meaning as one type of buffer.
2. Identifying religious coping methods associated with better or poorer mental/physical adjustment to stressful events, i.e., prayer.
3. Identifying spiritual coping techniques in the context of other means of coping.

The assessment process may also include consideration of the following:

1. Clinicians' potential biases.
2. Interview questions for assessing a person's use of religion/spirituality in coping.
3. Questions about assessing religious beliefs and behaviors.
4. Clarification of values.

The DSM IV's Diagnosis of Religious or Spiritual Problem

The American Psychological Association has established a diagnosis for religious and spiritual problems in sectionV62.89 Religious or Spiritual Problem. This category can be used when the focus of clinical attention is a religious or spiritual problem (American Psychological Association, 1994, p.685). Examples include experiences that involve:

1. Loss of questioning of faith;
2. Problems associated with conversion to a new faith;

3. Questioning of spiritual values that may not necessarily be related to an organized church or religious institution; or

4. Questions arising from near-death or mystical experiences.

Diagnostic Section in DSM IV

The American Psychological Association has also identified other conditions that may be a focus of clinical attention. The diagnosis is coded on Axis I and is related to Axis I and II diagnoses in the following ways:

1. The person does not have a mental disorder but "religious or spiritual problem" is the focus of treatment.

2. The person has a mental disorder but "religious or spiritual problem" is unrelated.

3. The person has a mental disorder related to the problem, but "religious or spiritual problem" is "sufficiently severe to warrant independent clinical attention"

(American Psychological Association, 1994, p. 675).

Differential Diagnoses

There are differential diagnoses possible based upon *psychotic experiences with religious content versus normal intense religious experiences.* According to Greenberg and Witzum (1991), psychotic episodes are:

• More intense then normative religious experiences.

• Often terrifying and preoccupying for the person.

• Associated with deterioration in social/self-care functioning.

• Often involve special messages from religious figures.

Dissociative Disorders Versus Normal, Relgiously-toned Dissociate

Dissociative Disorders involve "a disruption in the usually integrated functions of consciousness, memory, identity, or perception of the environment", which cause distress or interfere with occupational and social functioning (American Psychological Association, 1994, p. 477). Dissociative states are a "common and accepted expression of cultural activities or religious experience in many societies" (American Psychological Association, 1994, p. 477). Consequently, dissociation by itself "should not be considered inherently pathological and often does not lead to significant distress, impairment, or help-seeking behavior" (American Psychological Association, 1994,p.477).

An example of a dissociate state would be *Dissociative Trance Disorder*, which is a diagnosis for further study in DSM IV. Diagnosis is made only if the observed "trance state is not accepted as a normal part of a collective cultural or religious practice" (American Psychological Association, 1994, p.729).

Application to Social Work Practice: Ethics

Social workers and spiritual leaders can collaborate for the benefit of their clients. There are no ethical mandates requiring a separation of these two professionals. Ethical mandates actually promote such collaboration and come from the National Association of Social Workers' Code of Ethics. These ethical considerations fall into two categories: (a) social workers' responsibility to clients; and, (b) social workers' responsibility to society.

Section II (F,3) of the National Association of Social Workers' Code of Conduct reads:

> The social worker should not practice, condone, facilitate or collaborate with any form of discrimination on the basis of race, color, sex, sexual orientation, age, religion...

This provision against discrimination is broad in scope and prohibits discrimination across a broad spectrum of classes. This book breaks new ground for social workers, psychologists, marriage and family therapists, psychiatrists, and others in the mental health field in that it offers knowledge that can be used in bridging social work and spirituality.

Spiritual Interventions

It is wise to pursue a middle ground in attempting to modify destructive religious beliefs, such as those leading clients to:

- avoid reality and responsibility
- behave self-destructively (e. g., staying with an abusive partner)
- have false expectations of God (e.g., the promise of a problem-free life)

Here, the social worker can attempt to modify the "demanding and evaluative nature" of these beliefs without dismissing them completely (Johnson, 2000, p. 16).

It is inappropriate to impose the religious beliefs of the social worker upon the client, or to attempt to proselytize clients to join a particular religious group or organization. Social workers can be supportive of spiritual growth without becoming engrossed in doctrinal issues by interpreting spiritual growth in a broad sense. The social worker can assist the client in finding meaning in traumatic and painful events of life.

Crisis Counseling

A crisis can be viewed as either a danger or an opportunity. The impact of a medical crises, such as heart attack, breast cancer, spinal cord injury, impaired fertility, stroke, and chronic rheumatic diseases, will vary according to the clients and what meaning they make of the event. Psychological crises, such as divorce, bereavement, disasters, war, and combat, are also times when clients look to spiritual support in coping.

Research has shown that a majority of people find benefits from a crisis or trauma, a process which can be termed "meaning-making", "benefit-finding", or "post-traumatic growth"(Moos and Schaefer, 1998). On the other hand, a minority of people do not find benefits: they may "manifest long-term bitterness and suspiciousness" or may become locked into "ruminative thought" without finding meaning (Taylor, 2000, p. 105).

Preliminary evidence shows that for those coping with an illness, finding meaning is associated with better physical outcomes (Taylor, 2000). Examples of this are as follows:

1. Male heart attack victims were less likely to have a subsequent attack.
2. Recently bereaved HIV-positive men who found meaning in the loss maintained their CD4 T helper cells (a measure of immune system strength) over a 2-3 year period, whereas those who did not showed a decline in the cells and a higher mortality rate.

The most commonly reported examples of *meaning-making* after a crisis are:

1. Strengthening of relationships with family and friends.
2. Positive personality changes–increased patience, tolerance, empathy, and courage.
3. Changes in life's priorities and goals: "What is really most important to me in life?"

(Affleck & Tennen, 1996)

Spiritually Related Sources of Meaning After Crisis

According to Tedeschi (1998), there are sources of meaning that can be gained after a crisis is experienced. These are as follows:

1. Deeper connection with and compassion for others.
2. Facing mortality and greater acceptance of death.
3. Increased commitment to religion of the self-transcendent.

12-Step Programs: Addiction and Spirituality

Practically all American Indian alcoholism treatment programs utilize the 12-step program in addition to the traditional sweat lodge ceremony. Most American Indian substance abuse counselors view alcoholism as a disease of the spirit.

Social workers should become familiar with the spiritual philosophy of the 12-step program as a spiritual resource for clients struggling with addictions of all types. Clinicians may wish to refer clients to 12-step programs for gambling, eating disorders, drug and alcohol addictions, and sexual addictions. Tonigan, Toscova and Connors (1999) argue that "Correlational research suggests that 12[-]step participation is associated with reductions in targeted behavior, such as drinking, illicit drug use, or overeating. Likewise, membership in 12[-]step programs has been associated with improved psychosocial functioning and increased commitment to change, and it may offset the influence of unsupportive social networks" (p. 112).

The Key Spiritual Beliefs in 12- Step Programs are:

- Higher Power, or transcendent being: definition is left to the individual.
- Personal Relationship with the Higher Power: Because the individual is seen as powerless over the addiction, the Higher Power serves as the primary source of strength for preventing relapse. The individual communes with the Higher Power primarily through prayer and meditation.
- Miraculous intervention from the Higher Power so that sobriety can be achieved: The Higher Power has accomplished what the addict could not.
- Daily Renewal of Spiritual Practice: "spirituality has neither a past nor a future for AA members. In essence, spirituality is only experi-

enced in the present tense and may evaporate at any moment yet be restored as quickly" (Tonigan, Toscova, and Connors, 1999, p.119).

• Serenity: Acceptance of personal limitations and current circumstances. Epitomized by the Serenity Prayer.

THE SERENITY PRAYER
(author unknown)

God grant me the serenity to accept the things I cannot change,
The courage to change the things I can,
And the wisdom to know the difference.
Living one day at a time,
Enjoying one moment at a time,
Accepting hardship as a pathway to peace,
Taking this sinful world as it is,
Not as I would have it.
Trusting that you will make all things right
If I surrender to your will,
So that I may be reasonably happy in this life
And supremely happy with you forever in the next.

The 12-Steps of Alcoholics Anonymous (Alcoholics Anonymous, 1976)

1. We admitted we were powerless over alcohol—that our lives had become unmanageable.
2. Came to believe that a Power greater than ourselves could restore us to sanity.
3. Made a decision to turn our will and our lives over to the care of God as we understood Him.
4. Made a searching and fearless moral inventory of ourselves.
5. Admitted to God, to ourselves, and to another human being the exact nature of our wrongs.

6. Were entirely ready to have God remove all these defects of character.

7. Humbly asked Him to remove our shortcomings.

8. Made a list of all persons we had harmed, and became willing to make amends to them all.

9. Made direct amends to such people wherever possible, except when to do so would injure them or others.

10. Continued to take personal inventory and, when we were wrong, promptly admitted it.

11. Sought through prayer and meditation to improve our conscious contact with God as we understood Him, praying only for knowledge of His will for us and the power to carry that out.

12. Having a spiritual awakening as the result of these steps, we tried to carry this message to alcoholics, and to practice these principles in all our affairs.

Case Vignettes

To illustrate what has been articulated in this chapter, some case vignettes are presented in this section. These three clients examined their spiritual lives and were able to grow spiritually from their life experiences. They gained some meaning from these experiences and became stronger and more at peace with themselves after the social worker counseled them around their spirituality.

Case of Mary

Mary was a young single American Indian woman and a member of a California tribe. Her mother and grandmother had been shamans and had ministered to their tribe for most of their adult lives. Mary was having recurrent dreams of being called by the spirit to follow her mother and grandmother to a committed life of healing others. Mary did not want that responsibility and was torn between her own interests and what she saw as the spirit calling her to do. Mary was reminded by the social worker that she has free will and that she need not become a shaman, but could do the work of the spirit in many ways. After several sessions, she was able to get on with her life, as a contributing member of the tribal community, but not as a shaman.

Case of James

James was a young gay man, who was diagnosed with AIDS. He felt that the spirit was punishing him for his sins and that was the main reason he had become ill. The social worker was able to counsel with James and help him to realize that all of humanity are imperfect and all make mistakes. He was able to understand that his illness was treatable and not terminal. He was able to see that others become ill, and eventually all of humanity come to the end of their lives, whether they have sinned or made mistakes or not. In the process, he was able to regain his health, with new treatments and a renewed purpose in life, and has been working with other HIV clients as a case manager.

Case of Jane

Jane was a victim of sexual assault by a person not known to her. She was left to die after being stabbed and beaten in the process. She was overwhelmed with bitterness and hatred for her attacker. Although Jane never came to the point of forgiving her attacker, she was empowered by identifying him in a police line up and testifying against him in court. He was sentenced to a long prison term. Jane was able to tell her story in public gatherings of sexual assault survivors and spoke at hundreds of meetings. She dedicated her life to educating young women in survival techniques and volunteers several hours a week counseling rape victims.

Micro, Mezzo and Macro Levels of Practice

This chapter has addressed spiritual interventions with mental health clients at all levels. Spiritual interventions occur on all three levels of practice from individual forgiveness issues at the *micro* level, to 12-step program activities at the *mezzo* level, to work with community groups at the *macro* level through collaboration with spiritual leaders in the community.

Summary and Conclusion

This chapter has discussed *Spirituality and Mental Health* from the perspective of social work practice. Definitions of spirituality and religion overlap in many respects. Spirituality can be integrated easily into social work practice interventions. Ethical guidelines have been addressed with assessment and intervention techniques appropriate to clients experiencing trauma, addictions, and other problems of life. DSM IV diagnosis is discussed with attention to cultural differences and multicultural issues. Case vignettes are provided to enhance the understanding of clinical interventions. In addition, research outcomes are included regarding positive and negative outcomes from the limited research being conducted in physical and mental health fields. More studies are needed to assist social workers in providing spiritual interventions to a multicultural society.

References

Affleck, G., & Tennen, H. 1996. "Construing Benefits from Adversity: Adaptational Significance and Dispositional Underpinnings". *Journal of Personality,* 64, 899-922.

Alcoholics Anonymous. 1976. *Alcoholics Anonymous* (Third Edition). New York: Alcoholics Anonymous World Services.

Almond, P. C. 1982. *Mystical Experience and Religious Doctrine: An Investigation of Mysticism in World Religions.* New York: Mouton Publishers.

American Psychiatric Association. 1994. *Diagnostic and Statistical Manual of Mental Disorders.* (Fourth Edition). Washington, DC. American Psychiatric Association.

DuBray, W. 1999. *Human Services and American Indians.* Cincinnati, Ohio: Thomson Learning.

Greenberg, D., & Witzum, E. 1991. "Problems in the Treatment of Religious Patients". *American Journal of Psychotherapy,* 45,554-565.

Hood, R. W. 1996. *The Psychology of Religion: An Empirical Approach.* New York: Guilford.

Johnson, W. B. (2000). "Religiously Sensitive Rational Emotive Behavior Therapy: Elegant Solutions and Ethical Risks". *Professional Psychology: Research and Practice,* 31, 14-20.

Myers, D. G. (2000). "The Funds, Friends, and Faith of Happy People". *American Psychologist,* 55, 56-67.

Newberg, A. B., & D'Aquili. 1998. The Neuropsychology of Spiritual Experience. In H. G. Koenig (Ed.). *Handbook of Religion and Mental Health*. New York: Academic Press.

Otto, R. 1970. *The Idea of the Holy*. New York: Oxford University Press.

Pargament, K. I. 1992. "Of Means and Ends: Religion and the Search for Significance". *The International Journal for the Psychology of Religion*, 1, 201-229.

Schaefer, J. A., & Moos, R. H. 1998. The Context for Posttraumatic Growth: Life Crises, Individual and Social Resources, and Coping. In R. G. Tedeschi (Ed.). *Posttraumatic Growth: Positive Changes in the Aftermath of Crisis*. Mahwah, New Jersey: Lawrence Erlbaum.

Taylor, S. E. 2000. "Psychological Resources, Positive Illusions, and Health". *American Psychologist*, 55, 99-109.

Tedeschi, R. G. 1998. Posttraumatic Growth: Conceptual Issues. In R. G. Tedeschi (Ed.). *Posttraumatic Growth: Positive Changes in the Aftermath of Crisis*. Mahwah, New Jersey: Lawrence Erlbaum.

The Dalai Lama. 1999. *Ethics for the New Millennium*. New York: Riverhead Books.

Tonigan, J. S., Toscova, R. T., & Connors, G. J. 1999. Spirituality and the 12-Step Programs: A guide for Clinicians. In W. R. Miller (Ed.). *Integrating Spirituality into Treatment: Resources for Practitioners*. (pp.111-131). Washington, DC: American Psychological Association.

Worthington, E. L., Kuruso, T. A., McCullough, M. E., & Sandage, S. J. 1996. "Empirical Research on Religion and Psychotherapeutic Processes and Outcomes: A 10-Year Review and Research Prospectus". *Psychological Bulletin*, 119, 448-487.

Chapter 10

Healing and Communities

Wynne DuBray and Adelle Sanders

Communities, like individuals, experience trauma and are injured as a result of the trauma. The consequences of this trauma, whether it be colonization, national disasters, violence, or poverty, result in a "soul wound" (Duran & Duran, 1995). This "soul wound" manifests as post-traumatic stress disorder, which then permeates into the lives of the citizens living in these communities and is transmitted from generation to generation. Often this trauma never gets addressed and remains unresolved. In healing efforts, it is therefore necessary to focus on the community, while simultaneously working with the individuals who reside in the communities. Much effort has been undertaken toward healing communities, and this chapter will peruse some of these efforts, as an in depth discussion of community healing is not possible in the confines of the few pages included here. It is hoped, however, that through consideration of this topic—community healing—that those working in the communities of the world will become catalytic leaders in the efforts needed to heal all communities worldwide (Luke, 1998).

To understand the kinds of wounds that can occur in communities and what efforts have been utilized to heal these communities, we do not have to look far today. Communities, such as Oklahoma City, Oklahoma and Wounded Knee, South Dakota, have conducted prayer rituals and healing ceremonies in the aftermath of the loss of life of hundreds of their residents. In the case of Oklahoma City, the Federal Building was bombed and totally destroyed, leading to the death of many men, women, and children. Prayer vigils have been conducted on an annual basis to remember those who died and to come together for emotional support and healing. In the Wounded Knee Massacre of 1890, the Lakota people killed by the United States' government troops were mostly elderly men, elderly women, and children. Many were frozen to death after being wounded by the soldiers, as they fell to the ground in sub zero weather. For years, the descendants of the dead suffered from depression, grief, and other symptoms of post-traumatic stress.

Maria Brave Heart, a Lakota professor, developed a model to assist communities, such as Wounded Knee, in grieving their losses and bringing closure to a sad day in the history of the Lakota Nation. This model/theory of historical trauma evolved from qualitative and quantitative research, clinical experience, and observations among the Lakota (Yellow Horse Brave Heart & DeBruyn, 1998). Historical trauma is the emotional and psychological injury passed on intergenerationally that results from the genocide of Natives and the resultant ongoing oppression (Legters, 1988; Stannard, 1992; Thornton, 1987). This response includes, but is not limited to, anxiety, depression, self- destructive behavior, substance abuse, poor affect tolerance, survivor guilt, intrusive trauma imagery, identification with ancestral pain, fixation to trauma, somatic symptoms, and elevated mortality rates (Yellow Horse Brave Heart & DeBruyn, 1998). This generational trauma impairs natural mourning.

Even today, as this book is being finalized for press, a far reaching community experience has occurred that can teach us much about community healing. In New York City, the World Trade Center was destroyed by evil terrorists, which has created a "national soul would". Citizens throughout the entire nation are experiencing symptoms of PTSD to varying degrees. What is remarkable about this tragedy is what has occurred toward healing our nation. Throughout the country, Americans have unified and come together in various proactive steps to empower themselves and contribute to the healing process. In addition, various community meetings and prayer services have occurred–these services have actually stepped out of the bounds of denomination and dogma to a higher level of spirituality and unity. The clergy of all faiths have participated together, on one platform, and offered prayer and words to foster the healing of the "national soul wound". Through participating in rallies, prayer services, and community events, members of the society have gained a connectedness that has long been missing from the American society. In fact, locally, the suicide prevention hotline reported to the news media a drop in the number of calls they were receiving. Churches have reported increased attendance, and bookstores have reported an increase in the sales of spiritually based literature. The local news media reported that couples were even cancelling divorce proceedings. What is even more remarkable is that through proactive efforts, by young and old and rich and poor alike, the collective nation has raised over a billion dollars in less than a month from public philanthropy. This, for those of us who have worked to fund raise and develop resources, is an incredible feat to say the least. This all demonstrates that there is spiritual growth through crisis (Robertson, 1998). This also demonstrates what can happen when a civil society is whole and functioning (Wuthnow, 1998).

Examples of how communities can be healed, and how people living in communities have taken steps through empowerment to heal their own communities, abound. Whether this be a faith based community that provides mental health services in an African American church (Chatters, Levin, & Lincoln, 2000) or just the kinship that grows out of community in an African American neighborhood (Howze & Weberman, 2001), we can learn from what has been done. In predominantly African American towns in Oklahoma, the communities have established what they call "covenants of care" which have become important symbols of community support for elders that had previously received little or no assistance as they aged alone or within their struggling families (McAuley, 2001).

Another community improved access to hospice by addressing cultural and institutional barriers that existed in the community's service delivery systems (Reese, Aher, Nair, O'Faire, & Warren, 1999). Another community sought to heal family wounds, by addressing family violence in its service delivery area (Wade, 1999). In Tunica, Mississippi, with a $500,000 grant, the county housing group created a whole village for its housing project residents comprised of mostly African Americans; this village fosters home ownership for the residents and provides various social services (Jones, 2000). Ghettos and barrios have addressed poverty by matching residents to jobs with a great deal of success, which is empowering to the residents ((Elliott & Sims, 2001), while one community developed a "vocational souljourn paradigm", a model of adult development wherein spiritual wellness as meaning, being, and doing in work and life is the focus (Brewer, 2001).

The list of examples can go on and on, but what is important is that healing plays a significant role in community. It needs to be part of the community's infrastructure, as well as part of the community's economic and social development (Sfeir-Younis, 1999; Deikman, 2001). Communities can foster coalition building or competition, both of which have different outcomes, with coalition building facilitating healing (Evelyn, 1999).Communities can come together, as communities have done with church burnings in some African American communities (Carter, 1999), or foster isolation and alienation. It is the role of the community practitioner to foster and catalyze the healing of the community through using both empowerment and strength-based practice paradigms (Cox & Parsons, 1994; Rivera & Erlich, 1998; Saleeby, 1992).

Sanders has spent over twenty-one years working with poverty and indigenous communities in their healing processes and in tribal restoration and reconstruction. In this chapter, some of this work will be shared to the readers. In addition, in the context of the chapter a discussion of some tools that are effective to use when working with communities in their healing process is offered. Furthermore, some discussion is given about organized religion, spirituality in the workplace, religious conflicts in the workplace, and applications to social work.

Community Practice Examples

Sanders selected two examples from her many years of community practice to illustrate social work practice and community healing. Both of these examples will be briefly summarized. The first example is from her work with poverty communities, and the other is from her work with tribal communities.

Poverty Community

This community is a very small working poor community, with an incredibly diverse population. In this work, the tools used were empowerment theory, strength-based practice, coalition building, political systems, community planning, and leadership building. The first task involved changing the city council's perceptions of this community because it was perceived to be a community of middle class elderly, so not many social services were being provided. However, the community was actually comprised of a multi-ethnic, working poor citizenry. The next task was to build a task force of local, natural leaders, representing the diversity in the community. Once this task force was assembled, the community planning process began–the citizens, through using a nominal group process, developed a twenty-year community plan. The first activities included the construction of playgrounds for the children, street lights for public safety, and curbs, gutters, and sidewalks. The parks were constructed, and the group planned a multicultural community land celebration event, which involved the entire community. Because the next item on the agenda was speed bumps in front of the elementary school, and the city had rejected this as necessary based upon its traffic study, the task force put together a petition and letters to be signed by local citizens–they used the land celebration as a place to gather the most signatures. The group attended the next city council meeting and presented the signatures. They were then approved for speed bumps, but the city budget would not permit the construction for years. So the group got the work and materials donated from a local construction company. The city then approved immediate construction of the speed bumps because it had no policy to accept the donation from the construction company. The task group then ran someone for city council, thereby becoming knowledgeable of the political process–their candidate did not win, but from then on this community was active in all elections. This community has seen actualized many of their wants identified in their twenty-year plan. They now have a police station in the community. Now they are working on getting their community building. What happened in the community was self empowerment and healing, both of which have had a long term impact on this community and the quality of life of its citizens.

Tribal Community

Much of the work done in tribal communities requires what is called an advanced generalist perspective, because there are multi-systems and multi-layers of problems to be worked on simultaneously (Sanders, 2000). Clearly, tribal communities have been impacted by colonization and many, many federal Indian policies that continued to oppress them. One northern California tribe was terminated, as have been most of the California Indian tribes. This community began its restoration process with a law suit against the federal government, seeking to be restored to its sovereign status as a federally recognize tribe. Sanders began to work with this tribe at this time. The tools necessary for the task are: a clear understanding of social work practice across all levels–micro, meso, and macro; empowerment theory; strength-based practice; knowledge of court systems; knowledge of federal Indian policy; knowledge of culture and traditional healing practices; mediation and alternative dispute resolution; and knowledge of leadership, community planning, and local, state, and federal systems. Restoration is a complicated process. Once it is determined that a tribe can be restored, it is necessary to decide who is eligible for enrollment in the tribe, and a constitution must be developed and ratified. Both of these activities continue to oppress native people. The federal government determines which list of tribal members will be restored–usually, the 1950s termination list is used. This creates a problem in that only the members actually living on the reservation at the time of termination are listed, so this means that only the linear descendants of those on this list can become members. The problem is created when there are three siblings, but only one is on the list, because the brother was off in the military and the sister is married and living in town; these two are not listed on that list, and their descendants are considered lateral descendants. This means that they and their children, grandchildren, and so forth cannot become members of the tribe, unless the tribe sets a policy in its constitution to adopt them–this is detrimental to the psyche of those who must be adopted because it continues to make them feel as though they do not belong anywhere. Constitutions are another point of contention because the federal government has imposed the Indian Reorganization Act constitutional format, which is not often representative of the indigenous way of operating as a tribe, nor culturally acceptable to the tribe. In this day and age, many tribes are beginning to decolonize, and they are redrawing their constitutions to reflect indigenous customs and traditions.

After the ratification of the constitution and establishing membership, tribes in California have to acquire land, because most of these tribes lost their land due to termination–a forced assimilation policy of the 1950s. This land has to be placed into trust. The first activity that is done by most tribes is a land blessing or celebration, or a big time for some California tribes. This celebration uses indigenous healers to offer blessings for the land and the community. This is one of the first steps to healing. There will follow a long process of community planning, resource development, creating social services, building houses and a community center, and economic development. These efforts involve developing natural leadership among the tribal members and often mediation and alternative dispute resolution, as there often will be disagreements along the way that must be worked through in order to heal the community. This tribe in this example created a twenty-year plan, which was divided into three phases. The tribe has completed phase one–social services, housing, community building, and economic development. The tribe is in its second phase–diversifying its economic portfolio, building a gas station, restaurant, hotel, and museum. Phase three involves the acquisition of a major resort in their local area–this resort lies on this tribe's original land, and the members want it back. The return of the original land will culminate the healing of this tribe.

Organized Religion

The role of the church and religion has been to teach moral behavior and to create a spiritual community of connection and healing. The church is the home of many varieties of spiritual experiences. Some of those spiritual experiences are:

1. Conversion experiences where people accept a new way of life based upon some spiritual awakening are very common. Christians are born again by accepting Christ as their savior and embracing Christianity.

2. Visionary experiences have been reported in many churches, where people claim to see visions and gain guidance in their life from these experiences.

3. Possessions are experiences where people relate that they are mediums for spirits that come in and possess their bodies for good or evil. Evil possession has led to exorcism practices.

4. Unitive experiences happen during worship services and prayer meetings, where people report having a sense of oneness with the group.

5. Healing experiences have occurred for many individuals who report that they have experienced healing in mind or body in a worship service or prayer meeting. The Sun Dance of the Lakota is a ceremony of healing of both individuals and the entire tribal community.

Spirituality and the Workplace

The work place has replaced the community for many people, and it is a source of social activity and support systems . Growing numbers of urban employees are finding time for prayer, study of a religious text, or simply to reflect on their philosophy and/or beliefs.

Bound by the principles of Hinduism, Christianity, Islam, Buddhism, and other faiths, wage earners and supervisors alike are finding many workplaces a more welcoming arena for discussions of faith and values (San Francisco Chronicle, 2000).

As the soup is sipped and the sandwiches munched, spiritual nourishment is distributed around mahogany tables. This kind of atmosphere is conducive to humility and deference when conflicts and angry feelings arise between co-workers.

Northern California is a haven for diversity and a snapshot from the national picture. At a time when there is a decline, in general, in religious affiliation, there is an increased interest in spirituality. People are looking for some kind of coherence, in their lives, and wanting some kind of connection to others.

Many business leaders, in Palo Alto, participate in an economy that has fostered unprecedented wealth for thousands, but which at times is less nurturing for the soul. There is increasing demands on the time of employees, and stress can take its toll. This city in the heart of silicon valley is creating fifty or more millionaires a day. The employees, however, need time for spiritual nurturing. The focus of 21st century industry will be finding ways to balance work and spirituality.

Religious Conflicts in the Workplace

A balance must be found where individuals can appropriately practice their faith without imposing it on others. An employer has an obligation to create a work place that is free from harassment, intimidation, and insult. Government and business sectors remain divided over what constitutes religious accommodation in the work place. Corporate leaders have begun asking more pointed questions about how to help their employees infuse work with spiritual values. In most instances faith and work are not fully integrated.

Application to Social Work

Empowerment practice facilitates influencing institutions affecting one's life (Cox & Parsons, 1994). Events like the Wounded Knee Massacre, or genocide, altered this capacity to affect life and the government-regulated environment (Yellow Horse Brave Heart & DeBruyn, 1998). African Americans suffered similar types of oppression during slavery and during the civil rights movement as racism on the part of government officials altered the capacity to affect life and the government regulated environment.

Spiritual interventions for community healing is a new arena for social workers. Some have been involved in community healing work, such as assisting victims after natural disasters like earthquakes, floods, or tornadoes, by providing crisis counseling for individuals, families, and groups. Critical incident deprogramming is also a valuable service offered to individuals traumatized by acts of violence or natural disasters. There is, however, a growing body of literature on what communities have done to heal.

There are cultural differences in the way people resolve traumatic events in their lives. The community can come together and request the services of a facilitator, but spiritual approaches must honor the spiritual and cultural identity of the client, whether the client be an individual, a family, a group, or a community.

Ceremonies and rituals play a major role here, as these activities have the power to instill peace, security, and whole communities. Social workers can facilitate meditation groups and arrange discussions for employees in the workplace when employees feel a need for such activities. Social workers also need to become informed about the growing body of research on community healing in order to assess the tools needed to facilitate community healing in their social work practice.

Summary and Conclusion

Community healing is imperative. Negative life events experienced in communities have a significant impact upon the lives of the people those communities are growing (Young, Cashwell, & Shcherbakova, 2000). Spirituality, then is important to human health, as well as to community health (Spirituality and Health, 2001). Therefore, human spirituality must be incorporated at all levels of social work practice (Ackley Bean, 2000). Healing communities can be accomplished by incorporating spirituality into social work practice models at the macro level (Cascio, 1998). In final analysis, both community and spirituality are important aspects of culture, and to all social workers and human services practitioners working with people in the 21st century, culture does matter (Winter, 2000). It then follows that healing communities is a significant part of our work and should be paramount in our practice efforts.

References

Ackley Bean, H. A. 2000. "Human Spirituality in a Pluralistic Context". (Fall). *Academic Exchange Quarterly*, 4(3), 90.

Brewer, E. W. 2001. "Vocational Souljourn Paradigm: A Model of Adult Development to Express Spiritual Wellness as Meaning, Being, and Doing in Work and Life". (January). *Counseling and Values*, 45(2), 83.

Carter, C. S. 1999. "Church Burning in African American Communities: Implications for Empowerment Practice". (January). *Social Work*, 44(62), 7.

Cascio, T. 1998. "Incorporating Spirituality into Social Work Practice: A Review of What to Do". (September). *Families in Society: The Journal of Contemporary Human Services*, 79(5), 523- 532.

Cox, E. O., & Parsons, R. J. 1994. *Empowerment-oriented Social Work Practice with the Elderly*. Belmont, California: Brooks-Cole.

Deikman, A. J. 2001. "Mental Health, Aging, and the Role of Service". (February). *Harvard Mental Health Letter*, 17(8), p. ITEM01046002.

Duran, E., & Duran, B. 1995. *Native American Postcolonial Psychology*. Albany, New York: State University of New York Press.

Elliott, J. R., & Sims, M. 2001. "Ghettos and Barrios: The Impact of Neighborhood Poverty and Race on Job Matching among Blacks and Latinos". (August). *Social Problems*, 48(3, 341.

Evelyn, J. 1999. "Coalition or Competition". (January 21). *Black Issues in Higher Education*, 15(24), 15-16.

Howze, Y., & Weberman, D. 2001. "On Racial Kinship". (July). *Social Theory and Practice, 27*(3), 419.

Jones, A. 2000. "Little County Housing Group Creates A Village: Housing Project for Black Community in Tunica, Mississippi". (September) *National Catholic Report, 36*(41), 5.

Legters, L. H. 1988. "The American Genocide". *Policy Studies Journal, 16*(4), 768-777.

Luke, J. S. 1998. *Catalytic Leadership: Strategies for an Interconnected World.* San Francisco: Jossey-Bass Publishers.

McAuley, W. J. 2001. "Covenants of Care: The Symbols of Community Support for Elders in the All-Black Towns of Oklahoma". (June). *Journal of Aging Studies, 15*(2), 163.

Reese, D. J., Aher, R. E., Nair, S., O'Faire, J. D., & Warren, C. 1999. "Hospice Access and Use by African Americans: Addressing Cultural and Institutional Barriers Through Participatory Action Research". (November). *Social Work, 44*(6), 49.

Rivera, F. G., & Erlich, J. L. 1998. *Community Organizing in a Diverse Society.* Boston: Allyn and Bacon.

Robertson, P. M. 1998. "Through a Glass, Darkly: Spiritual Growth from Crisis". (November). *U. S. Catholic, 63*(11), 39-41.

Sanders, A. 2000. Social Work Practice in Tribal Communities. In Wynne DuBray (Ed.). *Mental Health Practices with People of Color.* (99-118). Cincinnati, Ohio: Thomson Learning.

Sfeir-Younis, A. 1999. "Development Assistance: Spiritual-and-moral-dimensions: Spiritual Side of Economic Development. (Spring). *UN Chronicle, 36*(1), 66-69.

. 2001. "Spirituality and Health". (January 1). *American Family Physician,* *63*(1), 89.

Stannard, D. 1992. *American Holocaust: Columbus and the Conquest of the New World.* New York: Oxford University Press.

Strasburg, J. 2000. "Faith and the Workplace". (December 14).*San Francisco Chronicle.*

Taylor, R. J., Ellison, C. G., Chatters, L. M., Levine, J. S., & Lincoln, K. D. 2000. "Mental Health Services in Faith Communities: The Role of Clergy in Black Churches". (January). *Social Work, 45*(1), 73.

Thornton, R. 1987. *American Indian Holocaust and Survival: A Population History Since 1492.* Norman , Oklahoma: University of Oklahoma Press.

Wade, B. 1999. "Heal Family Wounds: Building Family Strength". (December). *Essence, 30*(8), 42.

Winter, M. 2000. "Culture Counts". (Winter). *Human Ecology, 28*(1), 2.

Wuthnow, R. 1998. "Morality, Spirituality, and Democracy". (March-April). *Society, 35*(3, 37-44.

Yellow Horse Brave Heart, M., & DeBruyn, M. 1998. "The American Indian Holocaust: Healing Historical Unresolved Grief". *American Indian and Alaska Native Mental Health Research: The Journal of the National Center, 8*(2), 56-78.

Young, J. S., Cashwell, C. S., & Shcherbakova, J. 2000. "The Moderating Relationship of Spirituality on Negative Life Events and Psychological Adjustment". (October). *Counseling and Values, 45*(1), 49.

Chapter 11

Looking Back and Looking Forward

Wynne DuBray

Modern life has alienated ancient cultures, such as American Indians, Asians, and other indigenous cultures, from their ancient powers. In the United States, indigenous tribes were forced to go underground with their spiritual practices, as the Christian missionaries invaded Indian country. Only those who held fast to their traditions were able to continue their healing practices, which were based upon keeping in balance with nature, balance within the body, and keeping in balance within the community (DuBray, 2000). These healing practices were a basic part of the culture for thousands of years.

Western medicine, with a mere couple of centuries of experiences, is no match for this ancient wisdom. Western medicine is very expensive and focused on healing the sick and extending life. Ancient healing practices, in comparison, were very inexpensive and based on keeping people well. The majority of chronic illnesses, such as hypertension, heart disease, diabetes, arthritis, and obesity, in the United States, could be avoided by lifestyle changes in diet, exercise, and stress management. It is sad that more than half of the population in the United States, including children, are overweight. Too much time is spent watching television and playing computer games, while eating junk food and laying on the couch, instead of participating in physical exercise.

Modern science has given us the machines and technology to make life easier. For example, automobiles take us within a few feet of our destination, so we need not spend too much time walking. In addition, other appliances in the home free up time from doing laundry, cooking, dishwashing, and other time consuming chores. Furthermore, many working mothers, too tired to cook, stop by the local fast food outlet for their family dinners. These technologies and conveniences make life easier, but not necessarily healthier.

Recently, a survey was conducted to study lifestyles and health practices of the population in the largest cities in the United States. America's healthiest cities are Honolulu, Minneapolis, San Francisco, Colorado Springs, and San Diego (Gallia & Horn, 2001). The most unhealthy cities were El Paso, Tulsa, Houston, Memphis, and Detroit (Gallia & Horn, 2001). Categories investigated in the study were: amenities; physical health, environment; and, happiness. These categories were assessed on 37 criteria, which were then averaged and translated into letter grades for each city included in the study (Gallia & Horn, 2001).

The criteria on which the "amenities" category was assessed included the per capita number of acupuncturists, farmers' markets, fast-food restaurants, fitness centers, natural food stores, vegetarian restaurants, and yoga studios (Gallia & Horn, 2001). The "physical health" grade was measured per capita by rates of breast cancer, heart disease, obesity, smoking, fruit and vegetable consumption, life expectancy, lack of physical activity, and work sick days (Gallia & Horn, 2001). The "environment" grade was determined based on measuring air and water quality, the number of car pools, the politicians' votes on environmental issues, fuel wasted in traffic, recycling rates, and toxic-chemical production rates (Gallia & Horn, 2001). Finally, "happiness" was measured by: rates of crime, depression, high blood pressure, and unemployment; the number of charitable donations; the number of houses of worship; the number of surgeons; the level of poverty; the number of recreation areas; the number of road-rage incidents; the number of sunny days; and, level of traffic (Gallia & Horn, 2001).

We, in the United States, have fallen out of touch with our bodies' deeper rhythms and wisdom. We have become out of balance within ourselves. We can learn from the ancient cultures how to integrate mind and body and, thus, be more at peace within ourselves. The fast pace of a materialistic, consumer driven society is creating an unhealthy society, dependent on drugs for chronic illnesses and stress related disorders. In addition, many people self medicate with alcohol and drugs, such as methamphetamines.

It appears that people, today, are longing for spiritual experiences and connections, and they are looking for this in all of the wrong places. Spirituality is connectedness. We have become disconnected from humanity and the earth. We need to recover a sense of community and wholeness. Even though there is this pressing need to connect and achieve oneness with self and community, higher education continues to move further away and is not redressing this critical need.

It is unfortunate that higher education has become preoccupied with ego, pride, and money. The study of psychology has in many ways replaced religion for our society. Psychology is in need of change. Reductionism is being challenged. Reductionism created the lines of separation between mind and body, and it became superimposed over the spiritual domain as well. A paradigm was developed that separated God from Self. Anything of a spiritual nature has been considered as subjective, irrational, and usually ignored. More emphasis has been placed on spirituality and the Divine as being external, with less and less emphasis being placed on the internal (Seaward, 2001)

Human service workers can learn much from indigenous cultures by examining their world view, their view of time, their relationships with family, and their spiritual practices (DuBray, 2000). One need not embrace a specific religion, but can borrow those aspects of that religion which are meaningful to one's life. Each religion has something to offer. However, one need not be involved in any religion or organized group to find a spiritual experience or spiritual connection.

The wellness paradigm is ageless wisdom. It is based on the premise that the whole (mind, body, spirit, and emotion) is greater than the sum of its parts. Western science and academic knowledge are based on the Cartesian principle or reductionistic theory by which truth (fact) is determined by separating and examining various pieces. Much spiritual phenomenon cannot be studied scientifically. Spirituality encompasses the total being and is superimposed on all of life's experiences. This is emphasized in the work of a number of authors/ theorists considered herein.

Joseph Campbell

Joseph Campbell stated that all myths are clues to the spiritual potentialities of the human life (Campbell, 1968). Campbell (1968) further argues that our problem today is that we are not well acquainted with the literature of the spirit. Campbell studied mythology for over sixty years from the ancient Hindus to American Indian tribes. He found a pattern among cultures, as he studied their myths, legends, and stories. He also found in each myth that there is a hero. In his book, *The Hero with a Thousand Faces*, Campbell outlines the hero's journey. The stages of this journey include *departure*, *initiation*, and *return*.

Departure is separation from your place and family of origin. Leaving home is the beginning of the journey. *Initiation* is the road of trial. In every mythological story, the hero must demonstrate strength, courage, patience, and willpower. The *initiation* has two parts, after completing the test of life, the traveler progresses to a blessing of some kind. The *return* completes the story. The person on the journey is accepted by family and peers as an equal and benefits from experiences leading to wisdom. Campbell saw a connection between the rising spiritual hunger and the absence of parents passing on mythological stories. Information technology cannot replace the power of myth, and society becomes less civilized and more destructive.

Deepak Chopra

Deepak Chopra, a physician and endocrinologist by specialization, came to the United States from India. He was frustrated at the limitations of Western medicine (Seaward, 2001). He returned to his Indian roots and developed a series of seminars on mind-body-spirit medicine. His seven spiritual steps have been presented on public television and sold in video form to the general public (Chopra, 1994). His book, *The Seven Spiritual Laws of Success*, includes the following:

1. The *Law of Pure Potentiality* reminds us to enter in silence and get in touch with the core of our being, thus leading to the universal wisdom and the ability to create and reach our potential. We only need look inside to find our divine essence.

2. The *Law of Giving* is based on the axiom "as you give, so shall you receive". The law of giving reminds us to walk in balance.

3. The *Law of Karma* (or cause and effect) invites us to become more responsible for our thoughts and actions. Similar to the Christian expression "as you sow, so shall you reap", this principle encourages us to break habits that interfere with our growth and development.

4. The *Law of Least Effort* teaches us that the universe unfolds in its own time and place. To be in harmony with nature means to go with the flow and not resist that which we cannot change.

5. The *Law of Intention and Desire* states that we attract that which we submit to the universal consciousness through intention. We must detach and let the universe take care of the details.

6. The *Law of Detachment* is encouragement to let go of our desires, wishes, and dreams. We must trust that whatever the outcome, it is in our best interest.

7. The *Law of Dharma or Life Purpose* states that each of us has a unique gift and talent which we are to share with humanity. We all have a purpose for living and/or a mission.

The Dalai Lama

In his book, *The Art of Happiness*, the Dalai Lama states that compassion brings happiness. He encourages us to develop patience and tolerance as the antidote for hatred. He believes that the purpose of life is to seek happiness (Dalai Lama, 1999).

If one maintains a feeling of compassion and loving kindness, then something automatically opens in one's inner self. One can then communicate more easily with people and feel warm and open. One ultimately discovers that others are just like him or her, and one can then relate to others more easily.

Larry Dossey

Larry Dossey is a physician, who sees a new era coming in medicine in which the role of the human spirit is not only acknowledged, but also fully integrated into the healing paradigm (Seaward, 2001). After practicing medicine for many years, he was stunned to discover scientific evidence of the healing power of prayer. He embarked on ten years of research on the relationship between prayer and healing. In his book, *Healing Words*, Dossey has documented numerous research studies that have been conducted in measuring the power of the mind (which many consider the spirit) and prayer, which is a form of spirituality (Dossey, 1993).

Dossey provides a very thoughtful and interesting book on prayer, health, and healing. He describes how prayer manifests in laboratory experiments and how modern physics may be compatible with these actions. His writings speak to our deepest fears and concerns. He harmonizes the scientific and the spiritual, as well as the material and the non-material.

Summary

There are numerous writers in addition to the above that have introduced the spiritual perspective in different ways. Carl Jung's *Modern Man in Search of A Soul*, Maslow's *Self- actualization and Beyond*, McGaa's *Mother Earth Spirituality*, Neihardt's *Black Elk Speaks*, and Peck's *The Road Less Traveled* provide us with a wide array of approaches to finding our spiritual path.

The purpose of this chapter is to present a brief overview of some spiritual perspectives (Jung, 1933; Maslow, 1967; McGaa, 1990; Neihardt, 1972; Peck, 1978). These perspectives honor the divine mystery. We can study the consciousness, mythology, dream analysis, self actualization, prayer, and meditation to enhance our spiritual life. We can join discussion groups for spiritual guidance or organized churches if we so desire. We can take time to be silent and alone to reflect on our lives. Most of all, we can find time to find and follow our own spiritual path, so that each of us is unique.

Exercises

1. Of the theories or individuals you have read about in this chapter, is there one with which you can most identify? Why?
2. Consider Joseph Campbell's idea of the hero's journey. What stage do yo see yourself in now?
3. If you were reared in an organized religion, can you identify themes here that are similar to your religious experience?
4. Develop a plan to set aside time each day to devote to your spiritual growth and development.

References

Campbell, J. 1968. *The Hero with A Thousand Faces*. Princeton, New Jersey: Princeton Bollinger.

Chopra, D. 1994. *The Seven Spiritual Laws of Success*. San Rafael, California: New World Library.

Dalai Lama, H. H. 1999. *The Art of Happiness: A Handbook for Living*. New York: Riverhead Books.

Dossey, L. 1993. *Healing Words: The Power of Prayer and the Practice of Medicine*. San Francisco: Harper.

DuBray, W. 2000. *Mental Health Interventions with People of Color*. Cincinnati, Ohio: Thomson Learning.

Gallia, K., & Horn, C. 2000. "Lifestyles Survey". *Natural Health* (April).

Jung, C. G. 1993. *Modern Man in Search of a Soul*. San Diego: Harvest/HBH Books.

Maslow, A. H. 1967. Self-actualization and Beyond. In J. F. T. Bugental (Ed.). *Challenges of Humanistic Psychology*. New York: McGraw Hill.

McGaa, F. 1990. *Mother Earth Spirituality: Native American Paths to Healing Ourselves and the World*. San Francisco: Harper Collins.

Neihardt, J. G. 1972. *Black Elk Speaks*. Lincoln, Nebraska: University of Nebraska.

Peck, M. S. 1978. *The Road Less Traveled*. New York: Touchtone Books.

Seaward, B. L. 2001. *Health of the Human Spirit: Spiritual Dimensions for Personal Health*. New York: Allyn & Bacon.

About the Authors

Wynne DuBray: Ms. DuBray is a professor at California State University, Sacramento in the Division of Social Work and a Licensed Clinical Social Worker in private practice. She holds a Doctorate in Educational and Counseling Psychology and a MSW degree specializing in the mental health field. She serves on the California Institute for Mental Health's Cultural Competence Advisory Committee and the editorial board of the *Journal of Ethnic & Cultural Diversity in Social Work*. She has authored five books and several journal articles on multicultural issues. She designed and teaches a graduate course on Spirituality and Social Work.

José L. Guadalupe: Mr. Guadalupe is an Assistant Professor at California State University, Sacramento in the Division of Social Work. He holds a MSW degree from Rutgers University in New Jersey and a Doctorate in Social Work Education from the College of Social Work, University of South Carolina. He has held clinical, administrative, and program development positions in various fields, including family counseling agencies, drug and alcohol programs, and hospice settings. Some of his professional and personal interests include: on-going exploration into the mystery of the human spirit; human diversity and its complexities; and, developing and supporting programs and curricula that prioritizes people over profit or intellectual imperialism.

Peter Navarro: Mr. Navarro holds a Doctorate in Transpersonal Psychology. He has an impressive background in the healing arts. His early youth and adulthood were spent in Mexico, where healing is a common every day occurrence. He has studied and traveled extensively, researching the healing practices of indigenous populations throughout the world. He is constantly searching for mind/body connections that lead to the alleviation of human suffering. He presently lives in the North Bay area.

Sarah Rose: Ms. Rose holds a MSW degree from California State University, Sacramento. As a social worker, she endeavors to assist clients in spiritual growth and body/mind healing. She specializes in expressive arts therapy. She resides at Orgyen Dorje Den, a Tibetan Buddhist Temple in Alameda, California.

Marietta L. Rubien: Ms. Rubien holds a MSW degree from California State University, Sacramento, and she is a Licensed Clinical Social Worker. Ms. Rubien is an experienced family systems therapist and an expert in Brief Family Therapy. She has provided psychotherapy, training, consultation, and program development in the fields of child welfare and substance abuse. Previously, she directed an adolescent shelter, which developed and implemented family reunification, therapy, women's groups, substance abuse counseling, and after care programs. She is currently in private practice and specializes in "special needs" children. Ms. Rubien facilitates workshops on such topics as parenting skills, eating disorders, team building, and communication. She is a motivational speaker on self-empowerment issues. Ms. Rubien is also the mother of eight children, six of whom were adopted.

Adelle Sanders: Ms. Sanders holds a MSW degree, specializing in poverty and minority communities, and a BS degree in Applied Behavioral Science, specializing in cross-cultural human development, and she is completing her Doctorate in Public Administration at the University of Southern California, School of Policy, Planning, and Development. Ms. Sanders has developed an expertise in building healthy nations and communities and has extensive experience working in poverty communities and with Indigenous nations in their restoration and reconstruction processes; she focuses on healing and empowering these communities. Ms. Sanders taught social work for fifteen years at California State University, Sacramento. She has authored and co-authored many book chapters and one journal article on working with American Indian tribes/communities, and her dissertation topic is "Sovereignty and Empowerment Among California Tribal Nations". She currently is working with women who are both perpetrators and victims of domestic violence and as an Indian Child Welfare Cultural Expert.

Santos Torres, Jr.: Mr. Torres is a professor, MSW Program Director, and Pupil Personnel Services Coordinator in the Division of Social Work at California State University, Sacramento. He holds a Doctorate in Educational Psychology, Counseling, and Special Education and both a MSW and BS degree in Sociology and Psychology. Mr. Torres has presented papers at the national conferences of the Council on Social Work Education, the American Counseling Association, the Roundtable on Cross-Cultural Psychology and Education, the Western Social Science Association, and the National Association for Ethnic Studies. Workshop and seminar presentation topics include diversity, youth gangs, interviewing skills as a research tool, and school social work practice, programs, and policy.